THE ENERGY PARADOX

THE ENERGY PARADOX

WHAT TO DO WHEN YOUR
GET-UP-AND-GO HAS
GOT UP AND GONE

STEVEN R. GUNDRY, MD

with AMELY GREEVEN

HARPER WAVE

An Imprint of HarperCollinsPublishers

This book contains advice and information relating to healthcare. It should be used to supplement rather than replace the advice of your doctor or another trained health professional. If you know or suspect you have a health problem, it is recommended that you seek your physician's advice before embarking on any medical program or treatment. All efforts have been made to assure the accuracy of the information contained in this book as of the date of publication. This publisher and the author disclaim liability for any medical outcomes that may occur as a result of applying the methods suggested in this book.

THE ENERGY PARADOX. Copyright © 2021 by Steven R. Gundry, MD. All rights reserved. Printed in the United States of America. No part of this book may be used or reproduced in any manner whatsoever without written permission except in the case of brief quotations embodied in critical articles and reviews. For information, address HarperCollins Publishers, 195 Broadway, New York, NY 10007.

HarperCollins books may be purchased for educational, business, or sales promotional use. For information, please email the Special Markets Department at SPsales@harpercollins.com.

FIRST EDITION

Library of Congress Cataloging-in-Publication Data has been applied for.

ISBN 978-0-06-300573-0

21 22 23 24 25 LSC 10 9 8 7 6 5 4 3 2 1

To Essential Workers everywhere.
Let's get you some more energy, now!

control over your energy than you might think. We're going to take a good look under the hood and address this conundrum from where the rubber meets the road: the condition of your cellular energy system.

It all starts with understanding the three underlying principles that influence energy production and how to better harness them for a lifetime of health and vitality:

1. **You are overfed but underpowered**. Think about it. We have access to more fuel than ever before, and yet we feel out of gas. How is that possible? As you will learn shortly, the food we eat every day may look and taste "normal," but in actuality, it has a fraction of the vitamins, minerals, and other nutrients than that same food our great-grandparents ate. In addition, the sheer volume and concentration of "energy-promoting" foods we consume almost continuously throughout the day actually taxes our cellular energy system, which struggles to keep up with the constant onslaught of calories. We're going to look at why this is and how we can repair it, which brings us to #2.

2. $E = M^2C^2$. Inspired by Einstein, I created this equation to illustrate simply how our energy (E) is maximized. Now, I don't want to totally steal the thunder of what's to come in the following chapters, but for now, understand that M^2 stands for *microbiome*—the complex community of bacteria that mainly colonize your intestines (or "gut")—and *mitochondria*—the minuscule organelles inside your cells that turn the nutrients from food and oxygen into energy, adenosine triphosphate or ATP. If you have followed my work, you know that I subscribe to the Hippocratic truth that (loosely translated from ancient Greek) *All health and disease starts in your gut.* And as you will soon learn, your energy starts there too, because the trillions of microbes that reside in the gut

actually influence how much energy your body makes and how that energy is spent. Believe it or not, your microbiome and the energy-producing mitochondria that live inside almost all your cells have a long-standing relationship. Communication between gut microbes and mitochondria tells your body how to make and spend energy.

The C^2 in the equation stands for *chrono consumption*, my version of time-controlled eating with the right food choices. Eating the right foods within the right window of time gives your mitochondria and your microbes the optimal power to heal and regenerate. The result? Energy! Which leads us to #3.

3. **You've heard of probiotics and prebiotics, now meet post-biotics.** Your gut microbes and your cells (including the mito-chondria contained within them) communicate via compounds called *postbiotics*. These are gases and short-chain fatty acids that are produced when certain fibrous foods are digested by bacteria in the gut. Postbiotics constitute a newly discovered communication system between your gut microbiome and your mitochondria—one that is now under enormous strain due to assaults from environmental chemicals, improper and inadequate nutrition, and stress. In order to restore our energy levels, we need to restore balance to this delicate ecosystem.

But now to the good news—there's always good news, right? I'm the energy doc! You can absolutely turn around your energy production to make your energy equation work in your favor by attending to each part of the formula—the "Ms" and the "Cs"—and doing so in a manner that doesn't overwhelm your already exhausted brain. I'm going to make this simple for you. The pro-gram I'll share is a six-week process that meets you where you are now and helps you reclaim your health, step by step. No matter

CONTENTS

Contents

INTRODUCTION:
"I JUST DON'T HAVE IT IN ME"

Confession: I had absolutely no intention to write this book. The idea of writing about energy didn't fit into my plans. But then I received a phone call last year that I just couldn't stop thinking about, and everything changed.

I had been driving to a television studio in Orange County, California, where I was scheduled to do one of my favorite extra-curricular activities: appear on a fundraising segment for public television. As I got close to my destination, a phone call came in over the car's speakers. The producer told me that Kathy, a PBS presenter who was supposed to interview me on-air, wouldn't be able to make it in. "Did something serious come up?" I inquired, concerned for her and a little curious how we'd pull off the segment. The producer replied, "She's really sorry; she said she's been feeling like her energy has evaporated lately and today it hit her like a Mack Truck. She'd like to reschedule—she just doesn't have it in her to work today."

That simple phrase reverberated in my mind for a good few days. *She just doesn't have it in her.* As a restorative medicine physician, I'm accustomed to the majority of my patients reporting fatigue as one symptom among many—typically mentioned in a weary aside after a list of more pressing complaints. These days, about 70 percent of the patients in my Centers for Restorative Medicine in

Santa Barbara and Palm Springs, California, come for treatment of autoimmune conditions that have befuddled a series of doctors and specialists. I am never surprised that *these* folks—the patients I will always be grateful to for inspiring my first Paradox book, *The Plant Paradox*—feel like they're running on empty. After all, autoimmune conditions are by their very nature fatiguing, because rampant inflammation—which is both a cause and a consequence of autoimmunity—is exhausting! I've helped so many of these patients restore their health from the ground up, and in the process reclaim their lost energy, that I'm afraid I quite took it for granted that fixing the underlying causes of disease was part and parcel of fixing energy levels. Regaining energy was a natural by-product of fixing what ails you. *Energy comes back.* That inner pep returns. Call me an optimist, but I had always put more focus on the bounce back than I had on that inevitable low starting point.

But that phone call about Kathy helped to clarify something that suddenly felt bracingly relevant. *I've been an energy doctor for decades!* I just hadn't seen it that way, because that had been eclipsed by the more headline-grabbing stuff—the big-ticket items of cardiology, cardiothoracic surgery, and autoimmunity as well as aging and longevity—that take up more airtime in our current health conversation. The thing is, all of these health issues are intimately connected. Your baseline of energy, your resilience against diseases, your ability to live long and prosper—you cannot separate any of them from the other. And as the COVID-19 pandemic has proved, we can't take our resilience for granted any longer.

So while she doesn't know it, Kathy inspired me to start thinking more about energy and how we lose it. As I investigated the strange levels of fatigue plaguing people of all ages, it became clear to me that almost *everyone* experiences this unfortunate scenario to some degree today. I'm not talking about the sleep deprivation that comes after a night of caring for a newborn, or the woozi-ness that accompanies traveling across time zones, or the physical depletion that comes after a grueling workout; these are all situation-specific outcomes of unusual circumstances. I'm also not talking about the overwhelming fatigue suffered by my patients challenged with chronic fatigue syndrome, POTS (postural ortho-static tachycardia syndrome), or cancer—though for many, exhaustion is indeed a sign of underlying illness. The kind of tiredness I'm concerned with is the persistent experience of being drained of your usual energy, capacity, and sometimes clarity, within the context of your normal life. This is the hard-to-shake everyday tiredness that so many of us are familiar with but tend not to name—often sweep-ing it under the rug. It is a generalized inertia experienced by what I might call the "unsick," or as some in functional medicine call it, the "walking well." That term refers to those who consider themselves free of maladies—nothing's driving them to the doctor—but may nonetheless feel less than their best. Today, the walking well have become proficient at shouldering a pretty heavy pack of fatigue. And it's taking a toll on multiple fronts—from their personal contentment and fulfilment, to their ability to show up fully in relationships, to their ability to work, and to, I'm sorry to say, important aspects of their long-term health.

I started noticing this energy problem in patients who were see-ing me for general maintenance—keeping their vehicle in good working order, so to speak. They represented this new, slow-moving groundswell. These men and women don't have many diagnosed conditions per se, happily for them. They're doing okay by most assessments. Yet it's undeniable. An ever-increasing number of them admit, when I ask, that they are flagging and weary. It's not only the ones you might expect, like parents of young children, or busy entrepreneurs, or essential workers. Feeling exhausted is prevalent more or less across the board.

This phenomenon is growing in scope and reach. I notice it outside my clinic walls as well, sometimes in age groups considerably younger than mine. The friend who canceled a midweek dinner because the day had taken it out of her again; the parent at my granddaughter's school calling off the playdate because he didn't have the energy for it; the two mothers talking in the post office parking lot about how drained they feel. Folks, we are in the midst of an energy crisis—a cellular energy crisis.

What I've learned is that the reason you feel like you "don't have it in you" is because, well, you literally *don't* have it in you! Our modern lifestyles—from our nutrition to our habits to our movement and sleep patterns—deplete more than they restore. The result? We're constantly running on fumes. When our tank is empty, and we never refuel properly, we're bound to crash or stall out sooner or later.

With this book, I want to give "it" back to you. I will show you that far from being a figment of your imagination like one or more medical professionals may have told you (if my patients' anecdotes ring true for you), fatigue is a very real physiological state, and one that is intimately involved in your general health. After all, energy is what drives every cellular function. Energy is what keeps you alive. When you have less of it, your cells, organs, and tissues—including your brain—are at risk because they are being starved of the resources they require to function correctly. Unwelcome and disruptive though it may be, fatigue is a messenger from your body, delivering information about the state of things inside.

As I sometimes tell patients, feeling tired all the time is like being on the first curving section of what *may* become a downhill spiral. And you want to turn around now and scamper up to solid ground, while it's still easy to do so. Because there is hope—as I plan to show you in the pages that follow—that you have a lot more where on the diet and lifestyle spectrum you are starting from, there are ways to mitigate many of the assaults on your energy system, to restore balance in the gut, calm the immune system, redistribute your energy budget to the appropriate places, and care for your most important allies in health—your gut microbes and your mitochondria—so that your cellular energy system truly starts to work for you instead of against you.

As you may know, my life's mission is to get us human hosts to do a better job of the care and feeding of our microbial residents—I often refer to them as our "gut buddies"—so that these organisms can do the tireless work of ensuring we stay healthy. I'll teach you how to do just that. You will also learn how to repair and strengthen your gut wall, which will help banish energy-robbing inflammation for good. In addition, we'll work on creating the necessary conditions for your mitochondria to do their work of turning food and oxygen into the "energy currency" that funds the activities across your body and brain. By pulling back from excessive food intake and curbing some environmental assaults, they'll get a much-needed respite from being pushed to the brink. Then you will sprinkle in a little bit of *challenge* in the form of a unique type of time-controlled eating that I've used for myself and for my patients for the last twenty years that will further help heal a leaky gut and excite your microbiota and mitochondria into peak performance. Think of it as giving your cells—and your gut buddies—a proverbial kick in the derriere.

And there you have it: the recipe for reclaiming your energy. Doesn't sound *too* exhausting, does it? I know that when you're already dog-tired, your capacity for making big shifts to your lifestyle is pretty diminished. You need any changes to be easy, *underwhelming* (but over-delivering!), and to give you lots of small victories. You'll get them. This is no quick fix—it is a sustainable plan for sustained energy and vitality. The Energy Paradox Program is all about helping you understand the missing links to feeling your best and reclaiming the natural levels of energy that are your birthright. It may even help you reclaim your hope and belief in yourself in the process.

So take heart. If you're feeling demoralized about your low levels of energy, or if you feel that it's somehow your fault, I'm here to remind you that your body has an intelligence of its own and an extraordinary capacity for healing. As you'll soon discover, your body knows what to do if you give it what it needs and take away what it doesn't. Let's get started.

PART I

THE EPIDEMIC OF FATIGUE

CHAPTER 1

HOW DID WE GET HERE?

For years, we have internalized the belief that being tired *most of the time* is just part of modern life. I mean, isn't that why coffee exists? Being the incredibly designed species that we are, we humans are wired to adapt to changes, even hard ones. Plus, we have strong wills. When we start feeling out of gas, we try harder, pulling energy from *somewhere*. We reach for caffeine, sugar, or healthier "energy boosting" foods and supplements. We stock our bathroom cabinets with an arsenal of products to hide the evidence. (It's not surprising that a big trend in the beauty industry is concealer for men.) An attitude check—"What do I have to complain about anyway?"—may accompany the afternoon latte. And armed with all these reserves, we power through and get things done. Having studied and measured how we handle low energy for more than twenty years now, what I've heard from fatigued patients and readers of all walks of life is that they've learned to suck it up. Being tired much of the time is, they've told me, just a fact of today's reality.

I've got news for them, and for you: Fatigue you can't shake is not the sign of the times or the price you must pay for being busy or successful. It's not a natural part of aging despite what your peers or physicians may suggest. Not to toot my own horn, but as I am now in my seventh decade, my schedule is pretty darn full. I see patients six days a week, even on Saturday and Sunday, and I work at GundryMD, my online health information, food, and supplement company, every Friday. If I'm any indication, I *know* that being tired all the time is not a side effect of getting older or being busy. But I am not the exception; we are *all* fully designed to enjoy sustained, unflagging energy during an active, multifaceted day; sound sleep at night; and plenty of enthusiasm to start it all over the next morning. Having nudged hundreds of thousands of folks of all ages onto the Paradox programs (many of whom have much busier demands than me because, hey, my kids are all grown up!) and seen them reboot their energy systems, I firmly push back against the myth that fatigue is par for the course. It's *not*. The problem is we don't know how to talk about it, define it—or, as health practitioners, test for and treat it. It seems that we have normalized fatigue, instead of acknowledging the cost it extracts. So, let me reiterate: Just because you *can* push through exhaustion doesn't make it normal or right. And you most certainly do *not* have to live with it. As the poet Mary Oliver famously wrote, you have "one wild and precious life."

And if you've picked up this book, perhaps that's where you are too, ready to let go of the myth that tiredness is an inescapable truth of modern life. Maybe you're reading this in the middle of the night, wracked by another evening of sleep disturbance, or listening to it on your commute, pushing through mental fog to get what needs to get done, done. Perhaps you're "energy curious"—feeling more or less okay most days but wishing you had more of the mojo you used to have. Maybe, like some of my patients, you're at the end of your rope with persistent fatigue, and hearing an inner clarion call that *enough is enough*.

Some describe it as being too young to feel this old, or at its extreme, being downright wiped out. It doesn't matter exactly where on this spectrum of tiredness you feel you are right now; if any of this resonates, you're part of a very widespread modern phenomenon that escapes notice by most in the medical community but that takes a significant toll on individuals and on society.

When I started my restorative medicine practice more than twenty years ago, one of the most common medical diagnosis codes I wrote on patients' charts was, and perhaps not surprisingly still is, *Fatigue and Malaise*. In rare cases, such symptoms were the result of serious and life-altering illnesses, but much more frequently, I saw patients who suffered from milder, low-grade fatigue that can sometimes dull the mind and dampen the mood, and almost always drains quality of life. What might surprise you is that this second, larger group of patients, often coming for general checkups without any significant sign of disease, had identifiable, measurable markers of ill health in their bloodwork that were similar to the first group—not to the same extent, but still present. The very sick patients and the "sick and tired" patients are standing at two ends of the same spectrum of fatigue. I'm glad to say, the protocols I've developed have helped both groups—and those in the middle of the spectrum too—recover what they lost. Halfway into their programs, my patients are consistently amazed by the renewed pep in their step. It's as if they're suddenly recovering from what I call *energy amnesia*—a state in which their energy system was sputtering along for so long they'd forgotten what being fully energized feels like. With a nod to the cult 1960s novel by Richard Fariña, it's a case of *been down so long it looks like up to me*. Perhaps you know how that feels.

A Fascination with Fatigue

If you've been coping with fatigue for some time, you might be surprised that it took me this long to tackle the topic. After all, my whole MO is to bring light to the anomalies in health—the conundrums that leave most of us scratching our heads. In my previous book *The Longevity Paradox*, I explained why, despite the apparent increasing life span of modern-day humans, our health span is decreasing precipitously. In its predecessor *The Plant Paradox*, I laid out why, despite the adoption of a seemingly healthy and hearty, whole grain and plant-centric diet, many people continue to struggle with inflammatory and autoimmune diseases. (In case you don't recall, the answer is the improper consumption of gut-injuring plant compounds called *lectins* converging with a perfect storm of disrupters such as toxic chemicals and pharmaceuticals, causing leaky gut. You'll learn more about this, or get a recap, in the pages that come.)

Though those autoimmune diseases and longevity desires tend to get higher billing in terms of medical research than fatigue, I can't underscore enough that the ways we lose and gain energy indeed are the very essence of health or illness. Long before we coined more scientific ways to describe it, the father of medicine, Hippocrates, called it *veriditas*, loosely translated as the "green life force energy" that drives all living things. Having heard the same complaints of fatigue from people of all demographics, I've stopped taking this life force for granted. In fact, I've shifted this long-overlooked aspect of health—the functioning of your cellular energy system—from quiet supporting player to front and center star.

I realized there existed a glaring *paradox* I hadn't yet acknowledged, one that lies at the core of health, longevity, and disease: Despite living in a time when we are eating *more* energy-laden fuel than ever before, we are feeling more *deprived* of energy. We're living a much less physically demanding lifestyle than our forbearers, yet so many people are feeling physically depleted. It boggles the mind when you think about it. We're truly living in an age of plenty, and yet, we are plenty tired.

Traditional medical training quite frankly doesn't give everyday tiredness the time of day. This isn't because doctors don't care—most doctors and health care providers, just like you, are working hard under the burden of their own everyday fatigue. The system as it currently stands, however, is not designed to address issues that don't fit its paradigm. Medicine likes things it can measure and track; your energy level is not nearly as easy to quantify as blood pressure or cholesterol. One person's tired is another person's normal—there's no standard reference range for energy (though there *are* blood markers that correlate beautifully with your energy levels, as I'll share). For the average time-pressed and under-resourced practitioner, loss of energy is a fairly ambiguous phenomenon. And given the wide range of patient complaints, some physicians may even be tempted to conclude that symptoms are imagined or exaggerated—in other words, "all in your head."

Now, I don't want to throw my colleagues in medicine under the bus. But let's call it like it is: In the practice of modern medicine, if there isn't a pill for it, we often don't want to treat it. And if we can't pinpoint what it *is* or give it a fancy name, then how can we prescribe a drug for it? Given the sheer number of patients most providers are forced to see, the advice is, "Come back when things are bad enough to warrant medication or surgery." Sadly, what this means is that both inside and outside the medical provider's office, subclinical phenomena like tiredness; digestive distress; mild, persistent anxiety or low mood; and many other symptoms that drain vitality are never addressed. They're dismissed with a kind of "move along, nothing to see here" mentality—after all, tiredness is not contagious and, at least in a literal sense, not crippling.

Keeping Up with the Joneses

Of course, the medical establishment's lack of attention to the issue isn't the only reason why fatigue doesn't get its due. We live in a time of unprecedented expectations and few real safety nets. This forces many folks to push through the fog of low energy with a stiff upper lip, putting mind over matter—because if you don't show up for your family, your job, and your community, who will? Fatigue can also get shoved out of sight, out of mind in our competitive culture. When everyone *else* seems to be bursting with happiness and energy on social media, it can feel shameful to admit you're stuck in a much less picture-perfect place, scrolling through your feed with eyes half open. To make matters worse, few of us share honestly about what's going on. We're all too busy and too tired to listen to someone complain about being busy and tired.

But it doesn't have to be this way. First and foremost, let me assure you that tiredness is *not* "all in your head." It may *end up* in your head as brain fog, low mood, and loss of your old mojo, but it *starts* somewhere lower down in a place you can actually more easily influence—your gut. As you'll soon discover, gut-derived inflammation and microbiome changes are key drivers of this subclinical state, which, since it doesn't have a long name in the medical textbooks, gets a long name in mine. I call it, "When your get-up-and-go has got up and gone" or "get-up-and-gone" for short. (You can call it GUAG if you like acronyms.) If medicine isn't going to take it fully seriously, we might as well have a *little* fun with it.

The get-up-and-gone phenomenon exists on a spectrum from mild tiredness that persists despite following reasonable-seeming diet and lifestyle routines, to unpredictable moments of feeling like you're running on fumes, to full-blown exhaustion that significantly disrupts your ability to function. It may be untethered to any other palpable symptoms. But it also may coexist with niggling issues like poor digestion and constipation, hair thinning, skin sensitivities or seasonal allergies, generalized stiffness or loss of mobility, low libido, headaches, disrupted or elusive sleep, perceived candida or mold issues, and more. The good news is that I've treated patients across the spectrum, and even those facing chronic and severe disruptions to their energy were able to recover their get-up-and-go by following the Energy Paradox Program.

Stress, Coffee, Stress, Coffee

If you're thinking that the GUAG phenomenon describes many of the people you know, and you as well, you're probably right. I believe the overlooked epidemic of fatigue is a major issue—perhaps the biggest health complaint of our time. Statistics support this. One recent survey reported that more than half of American adults do not feel well rested on any given weekday. (While it's more anecdotal than scientific, when I surveyed the visitors to my own website, GundryMD.com, about what drove them there, the #1 answer was "need more energy" and #2 was "fatigue.")

A seemingly greater amount of data gathering has occurred on the incidence of stress than fatigue. This is equally significant, because stress and fatigue are bosom buddies; where stress exists, so does fatigue, and vice versa. Stress, burnout, and the resulting mental health issues have gotten more attention among medical professionals than fatigue, perhaps in part because of the toll it takes on employers and, by proxy, our economy. Fifty-five percent of Americans are stressed on a daily basis and eighty-three percent of American workers experience work-related stress (women report slightly higher stress levels than men). A recent large Gallup survey suggests that companies are facing a crisis of employee burnout, with almost a quarter of employees reporting feeling burned out at work very often or always, and an additional 44 percent feeling burned out sometimes. The *Harvard Business Review* estimates that this phenomenon costs $125 to $190 billion in health care spending each year.[1] It's not a surprise that an estimated 75 to 90 percent of disease states are considered to be stress related (stress begets inflammation, which begets disease[2]), and millions of Americans have sought medical help for conditions directly related to stress[3]—a number that has surely risen after months of COVID-related lockdown, remote working conditions, and the anxiety that has come with it.

One common denominator I feel certain unites all the stressed souls who answer the surveys: They're doggone tired. But here's a news flash for you. Over 95 percent of my patients who report feeling stressed at work and/or home and are overweight or obese blame their "stress hormone" cortisol for the fact that they are tired, bleary-eyed, can't sleep, and can't lose weight. Yet they have absolutely normal fasting cortisol levels on their blood tests. I hate to break it to them, but the issue has very little to do with the circulating levels of this single hormone in their bloodstream. That's right. I would bet that most people who think their problems relate to "high cortisol" on the one hand or "adrenal fatigue" on the other, in fact, don't have either problem (if you're shaking your head in disagreement, turn to page 61 for my take on why these issues are so widely misunderstood!).

The sneaky thing about fatigue and stress is that they sound relatively benign, but they have a large ripple effect. Tired and stressed-out humans tend to make poor diet and lifestyle choices that, unbeknownst to them, compound their fatigue. These choices include constantly grazing on food—thereby taxing, not supporting, their energy-producing mitochondria; filling up on "comforting" processed foods that starve their gut buddies of what they need to promote better energy; scrolling on devices after dark in search of distraction, inadvertently interfering with their natural sleep cycle; and even shying away from known stress-busters like exercise and connecting with others. The more tired we are, the worse our choices; the worse our choices, the more exhausted we become. It's a cycle that's hard to break.

To cope, we've become extremely adept at keeping tiredness at bay. We've come up with a panoply of substances to boost our flagging energy levels. The most obvious? Caffeine, a bitter alkaloid that, in nature, helps plants repel insects from eating them; in you, it helps repel waves of fatigue. No surprise caffeine is the most widely used psychoactive drug on the planet. Some data suggests almost 90 percent of American adults[4] and 73 percent of teens gulp down this stimulant on a daily basis.[5] Don't even get me started on the proliferation of teas and plants that promise caffeine-like lifts, the massive global market for chocolate, the decade-plus explosion of the kombucha trend (has it clicked yet that the reason this sparkling tonic is so addictive is because it's made of, well, caffeinated tea?), and the good old standby of diet sodas and energy drinks that deliver a buzz. You can all exhale here—I'm not inherently anti-caffeine. The problem is that relying on these quick-fix crutches masks the underlying issue: Your cellular energy system isn't cutting the mustard. But powered up on cold brew or Red Bull—and we all know how amped up that makes us feel—you never stop and look "under the hood" to find out why. That changes now.

A Global Quest for Energy

My fascination with finding out where our get-up-and-go got up and gone led me to revisit the research into the health of the Hadza people, a population living in the savannah-woodlands of northern Tanzania. The Hadzas are some of the last hunter-gatherers in the world, and as such, their diet and lifestyle has been extensively studied. Their way of life bears striking similarities to Pleistocene ancestors—they hunt on foot using bows, arrows, and axes and have no vehicles or guns; men hunt game, often walking 6 to 10 miles per day; women gather plant foods, walking an average of 3.5 miles a day. The Hadzas eat from their land, consuming a diet rich in tubers, berries, and honey during one part of the year, and during the other part, large game animals. They are remarkably thin and fit people.

The most remarkable insight we've learned from the Hadzas came from a study that aimed to understand the impact of physical exertion on the Hadzas' overall level of fitness.[6] Researchers wanted to test the hypothesis that this group of hunter-gatherers expend more energy each day than people living sedentary modern lifestyles, and that's why they are so fit. Of course, it would seem logical that all that walking and hunting and gathering ought to use up a lot of calories and ramp up the body's energy production. So, imagine the researchers' surprise at the counterintuitive results they gathered: The Hadzas' energy expenditure was almost the *same* as desk workers!

You might be wondering the same thing as me: Where is all that energy expenditure going for the desk workers, who by and large are sitting all day? Now, as researchers, when a study doesn't offer the data we expected, we still need to make a conclusion, even if it isn't a very satisfactory one. The conclusion of this particular study was that all humans simply have the same daily energy expenditure, regardless of their demands and activities. Perhaps this explanation satisfied some, but I found it too easy. The idea that an office worker's mental energy output rivals the physical efforts of a hunter-gatherer just didn't add up. I suspected there was another force at work—something that was causing unexplained energy use for the desk jockeys.

I thought back to my own forbearers. Growing up around my great-grandparents and their neighbors in the Midwest, there was a rhythm to their life. They got up at 4 a.m. every morning, had their cup of Folgers, and headed out for a day of manual labor or worked diligently at the homestead, raising families without modern conveniences and doing everything by hand. Nobody sat in chairs typing or talking on the phone all day and then pronounced, *I'm exhausted!*

Over my years studying longevity, I had observed similar phenomena, albeit in more bucolic, sun-soaked locations than my native Nebraska. Visiting small villages in the hills of Italy, I met some of the world's most vital nonagenarians and centenarians. In these places, the elders were still by and large living their traditional lifestyle, eating the same foods they'd grown up eating, following ancient routines. I was struck not only by their impressive health span, but by their extraordinary *energy span*; while most folks their age in our country find it hard to get out of a chair, the eighty-, ninety-, and sometimes even one-hundred-year-olds I met in Liguria and Acciaroli thought nothing of walking up steep hills multiple times a day, often herding goats and sheep ahead of them.

So why was the picture at home in the US so different, not only with the elderly but also in younger patients I saw who routinely complained of fatigue? And how could our relatively sedentary existence require so much fuel? It comes down to massive variations in diet and lifestyle, and a shift from exposure to natural forces (like full-spectrum daylight) to unnatural and disruptive forces like chemicals and artificial light—all of which conspire to change the conditions our energy systems need to operate optimally. The way I've come to see it, the average modern human is like a V-8 sports car that has lost half its engine power—it's running on four cylinders, not eight, and can't perform to its design.

The Hadzas, by contrast, not only had their original eight cylinders online and in great order, they had a supercharger on their engine and a turbocharger to boot. Their system is so finely tuned and well maintained, they're using the same amount of energy yet getting infinitely more output. Their energy efficiency comes from a lifestyle that keeps the engines of their body, the tiny power plants called mitochondria, in good working order, a clean-fuel diet comprising fiber-rich plants and lean animal meat, and a third important factor. They're avoiding the steady *loss* of energy that those living a standard Western lifestyle typically experience—one that happens via a phenomenon you're likely quite familiar with: inflammation.

ENERGY MYTH #1: A Viral Mystery?

In years past, the debilitating chronic fatigue syndrome was thought to be caused by the Epstein-Barr virus (EBV), a type of herpes virus. Many patients who have come to see me for help in treating this condition had "proof" of the diagnosis from blood tests performed by their naturopaths, chiropractors, and MDs. Consequently, when they arrived in my office, they were taking lots of antiviral tinctures and prescription antivirals and performing elaborate detox regimens—yet were somehow not able to shake the fatigue. While it's true that an active Epstein-

Barr infection in the form of an illness like mononucleosis can lay you out for months of bed rest (like it did to me in college), that's relatively uncommon. In fact, 95 percent of adults carry EBV in our white blood cells, and detectable antibodies to the virus are present in most of us. In focusing on such antibodies, these well-meaning professionals were missing the much more typical cause of chronic fatigue: chronic inflammation caused by leaky gut. Luckily, this is a condition that is quite straightforward to turn around.

Chronic fatigue syndrome isn't the only common misdiagnosis for persistent tiredness; because "fatigue" is such a vague symptom, I've found that many clinicians often identify an erroneous culprit. The naturally occurring fungus candida is often blamed for becoming an overgrowth and causing fatigue; the same with toxic mold or mycotoxin exposure; and even cases of chronic Lyme disease, blamed on long-term active infections of the Lyme spirochete—which leads to rounds of often devastating long-term antibiotics in the attempt to conquer the infection. While markers for all these issues may be present (and people have spent thousands of dollars to have them measured), let me assure you that association does not mean causation. Instead, I help my patients who are convinced that EBV, candida, mold, or Lyme are the culprits behind their lethargy to shift their focus. We get to work on healing and sealing the injured gut wall and changing the gut microbiome, thereby calming inflammation, thus reeducating their immune system, and this usually reverses their symptoms for good. What's more, over the years, I've heard from literally tens of thousands of people who, just by reading and following the protocols in my books, resolved these and many similar conditions that they thought were chronic and incurable.

CHAPTER 2

BODY ON FIRE

HOW INFLAMMATION STEALS
YOUR ENERGY

When Constance, a busy mom in her early forties, came to see me, she said she felt exhausted most of the time. She had been assured by both her gynecologist and her primary care doctor that as a working mom of two teenagers, it was normal to be wiped out every day. But when I ran her bloodwork, I saw that she had multiple elevated markers of inflammation. No wonder she was exhausted: Her body was on fire! Unfortunately, her doctors had not tested for elevated markers of systemic inflammation. Many—if not most—practitioners are still in the dark about these tests and, quite frankly, even if they did run them, they most likely wouldn't know how to fix the problem. Armed with this information, however, Constance was able to commit to following the Energy Paradox Program and resolve the conditions *causing* the inflammation over several weeks. The result was a return of the vim and vigor that she'd worried had fallen far out of reach.

The classical definition of inflammation is the body's "crucial response to microbe invasion or tissue injury to keep maintenance of tissue homeostasis." It is an ancient, lifesaving immune response that dates back—to simplify things greatly—eighty million years, long before *Homo sapiens* emerged. Your immune system's primary function is to protect the body from potentially lethal bacteria, fungi, molds, and/or viruses. It exists to swiftly detect any invaders the minute they breach the borders and then mount a defensive attack. That attack takes the form of inflammation. While you are sometimes aware of acute inflammation—the swelling of a sprained ankle, for example—much of the inflammation that is the most harmful to our health takes place outside of our awareness.

Inflammation really is like a fire; we need it to survive, but left unchecked, it causes damage, ravaging the body. Paradoxically, we now understand it's not the massive, ten-alarm conflagrations (like the body's lifesaving response to serious infections) that cause the most damage. Rather, it's the *chronic, low-grade* inflammation in response to the assaults of our modern diet and lifestyle that lays the groundwork for chronic disease. In fact, recent research has linked inflammation to just about every chronic disease that plagues us today, from cardiovascular disease to metabolic disorders like obesity and diabetes, to cancer, autoimmune disease, and neurodegeneration. The evidence is clear on this: Inflammation makes us sick. It also makes us tired.

Remember those desk workers who expended the same amount of calories as the Hadzas? What could possibly explain such a phenomenon? Well, producing inflammation uses up a *lot* of energy. And after measuring inflammatory markers for two decades in patients who don't feel particularly unwell, my conclusion is this: While the desk workers weren't exactly catching their dinner, their bodies were burning with the fire of inflammation—and maintaining that fire requires energy.

Cytokines, the chemical messengers that mobilize the body's inflammatory response, have a kind of executive privilege to spend energy where they see fit. This makes sense—after all, the body must prioritize survival above all other functions; if the immune system's defense forces detect a threat and need to mobilize, you better believe they will receive as much energy as they need! In fact, a number of studies has shown that inflammatory agents in your body actually *coordinate* energy distribution.[1] That means that when your body is devoting a lot of energy to its defense budget, there is less energy available to you for all of the things you need to do. Inflammation is a critically overlooked factor for people suffering from chronic exhaustion. It's been documented that even subtle increases in inflammation can be an underlying culprit in persistent fatigue.[2]

There's no denying it: An inflamed body is a tired body. So, you might be wondering, where is all of this inflammation coming from? If you're a devoted *Paradox* reader, you may already have a hunch as to the answers. I call them the "three Ls."

The Three Ls of Chronic Inflammation

The first of the three "Ls" refers to *leaky gut*. We'll discuss this condition in more detail shortly, but the basic concept is this: Thanks to a steady stream of processed foods, certain plant foods, pesticides and other chemicals, and overprescribed pharmaceuticals, the protective lining of our intestinal tract—aka our "gut wall"—has to weather quite a storm. All of these agents combine to degrade the integrity of the gut wall, causing microscopic holes to form that then allow bacteria and other harmful molecules to leak out of the intestines and into the bloodstream and surrounding tissues. Because 70 to 80 percent of your immune system lives in the layers of tissue making up the gut wall and in the fat that surrounds your intestines, *wherever there is leaky gut, there is also inflammation.*

If you had asked me fifteen years ago when I was writing my first book about my thoughts on leaky gut, I would have told you quite honestly that it was pseudoscience. But thanks to sophisticated tests now available and the work of numerous other researchers, like Dr. Alessio Fasano at Harvard Medical School, I can say with virtual certainty that leaky gut is an epidemic of its own, and can be found in the majority of the population today. Indeed, 100 percent of my fatigued patients have tested positive for some degree of leaky gut.

The second "L" stands for *lectins*, which are proteins found in certain plants that serve as their defense system to protect them and their babies (seeds) from being eaten by predators—including humans. Gluten is one well-known lectin—perhaps one you already avoid. Yet there are many others in legumes and grains—they're mainly found in the hulls of whole grains—and in some vegetables, like the nightshades, and in the peels and seeds of some fruits we call vegetables (like cucumbers and squashes), as well as fruits picked out of season. Conventional milk and dairy products are yet another source of lectins. Quite frankly, our modern diet is practically built on these pesky proteins (and, sorry, but most gluten-free foods are full of them!), and unless you are following one of my Paradox food programs, they're pretty hard to avoid.

As part of their attack strategy, lectins create holes in the gut walls of predators—so imagine the field day they have when they come into contact with an already weakened or leaky gut. Not only do lectins irritate the gut and cause inflammation there, but they're also able to sneak through the gut wall and into the bloodstream, where our immune system recognizes them as foreign proteins and triggers an even wider inflammatory response. I go into much greater detail about lectins and their relationship to autoimmune diseases in my previous books, but the key takeaway here is that lectins are *also* equally at play in the lower-grade epidemic of inflammatory exhaustion.

And that brings us to "L" number three, *LPSs*, short for lipo-polysaccharides. These are fragments or pieces of bacterial cell walls that make it across the gut wall and trigger inflammation, even without a leaky gut. I sometimes call LPSs "little pieces of sh*t" because, well, that's what they are. When contained within the gut, held amid the ecology of your microbiome, these tiny bits of bacterial cell walls are no big deal. But when they pass through the gut wall and into your bloodstream, they provoke a localized or even systemic defense attack by your immune system. Most of the time, the resulting inflammation takes place in your liver, which is bad enough for your energy production, but LPSs also can start cruising around in your blood and lymph, where they activate immune cells all over the body, including in your brain. Voila: a state of inflammation—and exhaustion—that never stops.

Unfortunately, there's another insidious way LPSs sneak into circulation. Research[3] shows that LPSs and even living bacteria can piggyback onto saturated fat transport molecules called *chylomicrons* and ride "through" the gut lining into the lymph system on the other side, circulating to lymph nodes (hot spots of white blood cells that catch pathogens to be destroyed) and to the liver— one of the most important sites of your energy ATP production. The ability of LPSs to make their way into circulation has led to a new understanding of why the standard Western diet—high in saturated fat—is so inflammatory.

Far from being something to muscle through or dismiss, fatigue is a *warning* from your body that it is burning with the fire of inflammation. It is a signal that it is trying valiantly to follow its innate programing and protect you from harm—but in many cases, you are the one unwittingly causing the harm. Instead of reaching for another double espresso, it's time to stop and listen.

Your Immune System at Work: Protecting You at All Costs

Clearly your immune system is the ultimate arbiter of your body's energy budget. In order to fully understand the role of this complex system in our overall health, let's pause for a minute and take a closer look at just how our defense forces do their essential work.

Your immune system is a wide-reaching network that includes organs, glands, lymph fluid, lymph tissue, and an impressive array of various immune cells that you mostly know as your white blood cells. Your gut plays host to approximately 70 to 80 percent of your immune cells. Why? Because your intestines are where the majority of foreign molecules—including potential pathogens—enter the body. Obviously these molecules can hitch a ride in the food and liquid you consume, but they also find their way to the gut in surprising ways—through your eyes, ears, and nose, and even your lungs (tiny hairs in the lungs called *cilia* push the offenders back up into your throat, where they are swallowed). Given this potential onslaught of bad guys, your gut contains a fortress of defense for the entire body.

What do those defense forces do? First of all, they scan for incoming trouble. If you've read any of the first four *Paradox* books, you might remember the "Star Wars early warning system" of barcode scanners called *TLRs*, or what I like to call "tiny little radars." They are found in all the cell membranes of your body including the white blood cells known as T cells, and they exist to look for patterns that indicate foreign invaders, mainly bacteria and viruses, but also lectins and LPSs that have escaped the gut. They also scan for friendly messages and proteins and serve as docking ports for hormones. TLRs constantly scan every protein that crosses their path—not unlike supermarket checkout scanners that read the barcodes on every product you purchase and instantly identify the item and its price.

Your TLRs have an important job: to ascertain if they recognize a protein or other foreign substance and assess its threat level—mild, serious, or nonexistent (aka "friend"). If a protein is deemed a credible threat to you, the TLRs immediately signal for inflammatory cytokines to get after them. These chemical messengers find the foreign protein, lock them in their sights, and call in waves of white blood cells to attack the invading enemy. It's an astonishingly complex but silently occurring process, wherein your immune system learns to read the codes of infinite amounts of matter entering into your body and gives precise instructions to the battalions of immune cells on the front lines so they mount the appropriate response. It's like a governing authority deciding if something is threat level one (a suspicious-looking package), threat level five (a missile heading your way), or absolutely benign (nothing to write home about).

Let's imagine you're exposed to the plain old flu. Your TLRs read its viral barcode, recognize it as foreign with the potential for harm, and say, "This is a bad actor; marshal the forces!" Pro-inflammatory cytokines flood the bloodstream to locate these invaders and trigger the first wave of defense—streams of sticky mucus to catch pathogens, coughing and sneezing to eject whatever it can. Meanwhile, signals are passed through cytokines that start calling in the heavy hitter forces—like phagocytes and lymphocytes, the fighter jets and missiles of the immune system—to directly attack the viral pathogens. And how do you actually feel while all this is going on? You're probably pretty wiped out. Your muscles feel achy, heavy, and sore; your energy is tanked, and you don't want to do much except watch TV or take a nap. In short, you feel like crap. But while you're probably cursing the dastardly flu virus for taking you down, the reality is you've framed the wrong guy. That little strand of viral material didn't in itself cause your fatigue and aches; your own immune cells get that honor.

While these adaptive measures are quickly being put in place, another even more fundamental imperative is put in play: a redistribution of energy. Your immune system *wants* you to binge-watch your favorite show or snooze on the couch. You are at war, and the frontline troops, your white blood cells, need all the energy they can get. Which means those back on the home front have to ration. Since your muscles are normally big energy hogs, your own inflammatory messengers make it hurt to move. Result: You won't use those muscles much, and more fuel can be allocated to the troops. Ditto with productive, high-functioning mental work; that takes energy too! Cue the brain fog and dulled thinking (we'll get to that particular pleasure in Chapter 5). No point flipping open the laptop today! You will need to rest. But it's in aid of a worthy cause: The troops are being supplied with as much fuel as possible, and the immune system rules the day.

Starved of Oxygen, You're Pooped

One rarely discussed nuance of our personal energy crisis is the way that chronic inflammation starves your cellular energy system of the oxygen and nutrients it needs to make energy. Inflammation constricts and stiffens the blood vessels, restricting the flow of those essential supply materials to your cells, thereby depriving your energy-making mitochondria of needed resources. I measure the "flexibility" of my fatigued patients' blood vessels using a test called the EndoPAT—which temporarily restricts blood flow in the arm using a blood pressure cuff, then detects how well the blood vessels spring back open even wider after the cuff is deflated, allowing extra flow to make up for the lack. When chronic inflammation is present, the springing back is paltry because the vessels' ability to dilate or expand has been lost.

As a way of understanding how this test works, imagine a car accident closing down the interstate, creating a backup of traffic. When the accident is cleared, wouldn't it be great if the four-lane freeway magically increased to eight lanes to allow all of those waiting cars to move more quickly? That's what your blood vessels should normally do anytime you need more blood flow. (As an aside, if your doctor tells you that you need vasodilator drugs—"Vaso" = vessel, "dilate" = open—including Viagra, what they should be telling you is that your system is rife with inflammation and let's find out why.) Inflammation around your arteries and resulting oxygen restriction causes a chronic bottleneck in energy traffic management. The good news is that by following the program in this book, along with taking a few simple supplements to lessen inflammation, you can help your blood vessels regain much of their energy-giving flexibility.[4]

Your body's brief viral battle tends to last a few days until pathogens are essentially "eaten up" and destroyed. With the invaders under control, *anti*-inflammatory cytokines now turn off the alarms, call back the troops to home base, and let the body know the battle is over—a state of balance, or homeostasis, is more or less restored. Good news for the rest of the body: The rationing is over and normal energy production and distribution can resume. Gradually you "come back to life," and begin to feel like yourself again. It's been a wild ride, but you are safe and back in action.

A disturbance to homeostasis, a flurry of activity, some concomitant tiredness, and then a return to the status quo—this is how things should play out after the immune system has launched an inflammatory attack. Yet what's occurring in today's epidemic of chronic inflammation is much different. The four-day battle becomes a never-ending war—the hatches stay battened, the fatigue, torpor, and brain fog persist, almost as if it's a flu you just can't shake. (In fact, we are now seeing this very phenomenon in some patients who have had the COVID-19 virus, called "long-haulers," who suffer a post-viral syndrome of fatigue, depression, and brain fog.) Over time, chronic inflammation can become your "new normal." You might become accustomed to living with a lack of get-up-and-go (sometimes accompanied by symptoms like brain fog, headache, heightened anxiety, weight gain, food sensitivities, and so on). And because it's a generally silent process, you grit your teeth and do your best to move forward while confounded—and sometimes quite miserable—about what's holding you back. Seen through my clinical lens, however, it's not such a mystery.

My patient Linda is one of many who have solved the silent inflammation conundrum. Linda was in her early fifties when she first visited my clinic, and I must admit, her markers of inflammation were rather impressive—and not in a good way. Interestingly, fatigue wasn't something she complained about in her appointment. Yet when she came in to review follow-up bloodwork after faithfully following the Energy Paradox Program to the letter for three months, I barely recognized her: A whole new person stood in front of me. "Doc, what's happened to me?" she exclaimed. "Suddenly every day feels like a great day—and I have so much more energy that I don't even drink coffee anymore!" As we reviewed her test results, I pointed out that her hs-CRP level, a generalized marker of inflammation that ideally should be less than 1—and which used to be at 10 for Linda—was now at 2! (I often refer to CRP as "crap," and not for nothing—when it's elevated and inflammation is running rampant, you do feel like crap!) It was no mystery to me why she felt so much better.

Seeing the dramatic change documented on paper, Linda laughed. "I thought I'd just had some kind of magical attitude adjustment. But obviously this change is real!" Linda is proof that when you reduce inflammation (as measured by that CRP marker dropping in her case), you'll begin to feel significantly more upbeat.

Achieving a turnaround like Linda's is always something to celebrate. Because if inflammation is left to smolder unchecked, it can lead to serious problems. At its worst, the storm of war, initiated by chronic leaky gut, can result in autoimmune disorders, which are rampant today. Autoimmunity is the umbrella term for the vast array of conditions in which the immune system becomes *so* hyper-activated that it begins to take aim inadvertently at "the wrong guy"—fairly innocent foods for example, or proteins in your tissues that are molecularly similar in composition to some of those foods—attacking and damaging them with often devastating results. This phenomenon of the immune system acting on cases of mistaken identity, termed *molecular mimicry* by my colleague Loren Cordain, is the ultimate example of friendly fire: The body attacks itself! Imagine the collateral damage this kind of chaos causes to your joints, tissues, nerves, and brain over time—and the amount of energy your body's armed forces use up in the process. It's my personal opinion that once we are able to clinically identify a few more very specific inflammatory markers, the chronic, lower-grade systemic inflammation that so many people live with will also be categorized as an autoimmune condition.

By now, you may be wondering *how* to create the conditions in your body that tamp down on inflammation and keep it under check. We're going to get there, but first we need to take a deeper dive into *why* silent and tiring inflammation is so ubiquitous today. It starts where the story almost always does today: in your gut and with the state of what I call your "roots and soil."

ENERGY MYTH #2: **The Key to More Energy Is Eating Anti-inflammatory Foods and Spices**

Many of my patients have shared with me that they've put themselves on an "anti-inflammatory diet," having filled their kitchens with herbs and spices, supplements, and bone broth and collagen powders, all touted to reduce inflammation. Invariably, these patients are confounded when their inflammatory symptoms don't seem to resolve. Why, they ask me, is their body still so inflamed when they've been diligently swallowing supplements and making broth and smoothies?

The fact is, in the battle against chronic inflammation, adding turmeric to your afternoon latte or throwing ginger into your smoothie is a bit like fighting a wildfire with a garden hose: It quiets the flames in a small corner of the neighborhood while the surrounding acreage burns down. If you have a leaky gut, no amount of powders and potions can compensate for the fact that the all-important border wall is crying out to be "sealed and healed" so that your immune system's inflammatory response can switch itself off. Healing leaky gut and restoring the balance of your microbiome is always where we need to focus our efforts to quell inflammation—which requires a more comprehensive overhaul of your nutrition and lifestyle than simply adding some herbs and spices to your diet. And frankly, there is scant literature to support that any of these anti-inflammatory substances can heal the gut. By all means, include these wonderful "extras" in your diet for their *many* health-giving benefits, but don't depend on them alone to stop inflammation in its tracks.

CHAPTER 3

DAMAGED ROOTS, DEGRADED SOIL, AND THE POSTBIOTIC CONUNDRUM

The alarming fact is that foods—fruits, vegetables, and grains—now being raised on millions of acres of land that no longer contains enough of certain needed nutrients, are starving us—no matter how much we eat of them.

—U.S. Senate document 74-264 (1936)

When I'm lecturing to physicians in the US, I like to show a slide with the quote above, without the source and date, and ask my audience when they think this statement was made. Most people offer a guess somewhere in the twenty-first century—some may go as far back as 1980. But no one has ever guessed 1936! Yet we have known for eighty-five years that everything is amiss in the soil in which our food is grown. As a consequence of modern agricultural practices—including the routine use of biocides and intensive monocropping—our soil has become depleted of the nutrients and the complex ecosystem of microbes that confer its life-giving properties. The plants we grow in it have gotten weaker, less resilient, and less nutritious as a result.

These issues are mirrored in our internal ecology as well. Just as the degradation of our soil is depleting our food of vital nutrients, the degradation of our microbiome—and its structural support, the gut wall—is depleting our body of the essential ingredients it needs for health and energy production.

As I was writing this chapter, a perfect analogy was unfolding right before my eyes. Outside my house on the edge of my yard, two hedges stand in close proximity. Each received the same amount of sunlight, faced the same direction, and received the same amount of water. Yet one hedge was sturdy and vital, with glossy green leaves, while the other withered, dropped its leaves, and looked quite pathetic indeed. My wife and I tried everything to turn this unfortunate situation around, using every natural soil conditioner we could find. Until one day I looked at the hedge as if it were a patient of mine. *Aha!* I thought. *I'm missing the obvious. I need to look under the surface and check the roots.* Sure enough, after a little careful poking around, I discovered that a crew of hungry, tunneling gophers had burrowed toward the stricken plants and nibbled away at their buried roots. With the roots under constant attack, the poor hedge couldn't uptake nutrients from the soil or enough water. Furthermore, the built-in protection of its rhizosphere—the complex and diverse bacterial community that surrounded the roots—was lost. In essence the hedge's immune system and roots were highly compromised, and not only was it undernourished, it couldn't withstand pathogenic bacteria and fungi coexisting in the soil either.

This is not too different from what's happening inside of you—minus the gophers, hopefully. Buried in the unseen world of your gut, you have an intricate system of intestinal "roots" for absorbing nutrients and generating immune responses. This huge system—just wait for how big it is—is brilliantly constructed, yet it can also be easily harmed. One of the prerequisites to do its job?

Lots of healthy soil surrounding its every nook and cranny. That's right, I said soil! You don't actually have loamy *earth* inside your intestines, of course; but you do have an extraordinary ecosystem of microbes, including at least a hundred trillion bacteria, living around your roots, directly feeding into your energy and health. And just like I found out with my hedge, when the gardener (or the U.S. Senate) fails to tend to the roots or the soil, or lets them sink into disrepair, the plant, like you, begins to droop, lose its power, and ultimately decline.

In my hedge's case, all was soon resolved. Once the problem was isolated, a little sweaty digging, a roll of chicken wire sunk in deep into the earth, a commitment to "rebuild the soil" using extra compost, and voila: The pesky critters were outwitted, the soil got richer and more protective, and the hedge's health began to turn around.

This lesson from the plant kingdom is important. You are not *that* different from your plant friends, because like them you are absolutely reliant on the conditions of your "underground" ecosystem, your soil, to grow and thrive. In this chapter you will learn to see yourself as somewhat plantlike (albeit a plant that walks—*you* don't have to be rooted in one place!). You'll discover your intestines' *microvilli*, the literal rootlike projections that dramatically increase the surface area of your gut wall. And you'll learn to lovingly tend to the soil that they are embedded into: That's the rich organic matter formed by the microbes that live inside your intestines, along with the proper food (let's call it your mulch) that mixes with them, changing by the day.

Gut Buddies: Your Soil's Superorganism

For decades, most doctors thought the intestinal tract was just a hollow tube with a fairly banal job. It took in proteins, fats, and carbohydrates; digested and absorbed them; and then waste products came out your rear end. (Just as an aside, this thinking fostered the now repudiated but still persistent belief of "calories in = calories out," providing the foundation for the useless weight-loss strategy of "eat less, move more.")

Now we know differently—far from banal or empty, your gastro-intestinal system contains a thriving universe of species that have taken up residence in this quiet, protected home, and that work every day to ensure your body (their home) performs optimally. This combined collection of many trillions of minute microbial organisms—bacteria along with viruses, yeasts, and other fungi, protozoa, and even worms!—collectively form your *holobiome* (though the word *microbiome* tends to be used interchangeably). These microorganisms live, barely noticed by you, inside *all* the places your body interfaces with the outside world: not only in your intestinal tract but also in your mouth and nose, on your skin, in your urogenital tracts, and, if you're female, in your vaginal canal and your breast ducts. Some of them even occupy your immediate airspace, forming a kind of invisible cloud around your body! (Imagine Pig-Pen in the *Peanuts* cartoon strip.) All told, your holobiome totals about five pounds in total mass, making it what some call a "virtual organ."

Why is it virtual, you might ask? Because, astoundingly, this very significant part of your physiology is not actually made of your own cells or genes. It is a massive community of organisms that have DNA distinct from your own and that work in a symbiotic relationship with your cells and your genes. This gives them something of a hallowed status in terms of your physiology. With its extraordinary volume of different microbial species and strains, your holobiome's cumulative genome is actually much bigger and more active than your own relatively paltry human genome—no offense. In fact, your holobiome is now widely regarded as a "second genome," enhancing and radically amplifying the work of the first one (yours). I imagine it as your always-available "cloud computer," sending and receiving information from your environment and your body, constantly processing data about what's going on, what's changing, and what's needed for survival, and sending messages back to your human cells. As weird as it sounds, your holobiome is where much of the real action is when it comes to your energy and health.

Of all the microbes that make up the holobiome, we know most about bacteria. Thanks to the Human Microbiome Project, a National Institutes of Health initiative dedicated to understanding the biome and its role in health and disease, we've been able to identify roughly one hundred *trillion* bugs, including ten thousand distinct species of bacteria alone. That's a lot of bugs! The majority of them—up to 70 percent—live in your intestines, and of those, we know most about the ones in your large intestine (colon). (Researchers are able to study the microbial composition of the large intestine because stool samples are fairly easy to acquire. Gaining access to the microbes in the small intestine, one step farther upstream, is not nearly so easy, making it the next frontier.) These bugs make up the ecosystem typically referred to as your gut microbiome—the health of which, as we've already discussed, is paramount to *your* health and your energy production.

Codependent Relationships (of the Good Kind)

The strains of bacteria and fungi that make their home in your gut need each other around—just like those in the soil of your garden. They coexist in an intricate ecosystem, one that's likely far more complex than even the most profuse rain forest on earth, with the activities of one species supporting the activities of another. When you have a healthy microbiome, the strains that exert the most benefit—your gut buddies—occupy the majority of the gut wall real estate, snuggled into a layer of mucus that lines the wall. When your helpful gut buddies thrive, it ensures that the occupants that can harm you—like the yeast candida, as well as the bugs that can cause serious or even deadly infection, like *C. difficile*—are kept in check. You see, none of the bacteria or fungi in your microbiome are inherently out to get you or cause you harm. Most microbes in the gut do have a purpose and a place in the system. But to keep good order, the most helpful ones— your gut buddies—should "crowd out" less helpful strains so they occupy only a small niche in the whole. This ensures the potentially problematic members of the community don't get a strong foothold or hijack your gut environment, taking it over and causing mayhem. And what this means for you as the "host" organism is that if you maintain the conditions your microbiome needs, this complex ecosystem of microbes returns the favor, taking good care of you.

The problems happen when you don't hold up your end of the deal. Starve this ecosystem of the nutrients it needs or bombard it with things it doesn't need (such as the Energy Disruptors on page 150), and the same critters that once helped you thrive can start to lose their power. Even subtle shifts in your microbial species ratio can throw a wrench into your health. Research has shown that changes in the ratio of two prevalent strains of bacteria (*Firmicutes* to *Bacteroides*) can negatively impact metabolism and lead to symptoms of type 1 and 2 diabetes, colitis, and obesity.[1] And when the balance of your ecosystem gets completely thrown out of whack and the less desirable bacteria take over the place, real chaos ensues. For example, your gut buddies produce a metabolite called *succinate*, which plays a vital role in energy production.[2] When the less desirable bacteria are in charge, succinate switches teams in a sense—it becomes destructive. It gets generated in excess, and begins to work as a counteragent, sending messages to your immune system to stay inflamed, while also driving increased fat storage.

When you envision these many, many strains all interacting within your gut, it's easier to understand why those of us studying the developed world's decline in health—and energy levels—over the last few decades are deeply concerned by the collapse of our microbiome's natural diversity. (Similar to the concerns of those studying our farmlands and global food supply, as the loss of diverse and thriving soil microbes is turning once-rich soil to "dead" dirt.) As we know from all types of ecosystems, when one species is wiped out, another loses what it needs to survive. The ripple effect becomes devastating. For example, the Hadzas, along with other hunter-gatherers who have been studied, embody microbiome balance at its best: Their inner ecosystem has been shown to be extremely diverse and "dynamic"—meaning the biome changes its composition in response to its environment, such as the seasonal changes that make different foods available. By contrast, the average Western microbiome, raised on processed foods, lacking in the fibrous foods our gut buddies need to thrive, and riddled with chemicals and stress, is as barren and still as a desert![3]

Your Gut Buddies and You: A Love Story

You may already be familiar with the shared origin story of how we humans came to host colonies of microbial friends. If not, a quick review to catch you up: Approximately two billion years ago, certain bacteria were engulfed (whole) by other organisms, and in exchange for food, they produced energy in the form of adenosine triphosphate (ATP). These engulfed bacteria became mitochondria. From this, the eukaryotic cell—the basis of all plant and animal life—was formed.

Now let's fast-forward a few billion years to when an oxygen-rich atmosphere developed on earth. Many bacteria are obligate anaerobes, meaning they cannot tolerate oxygen. (Think vampires unable to tolerate sunlight.) Eventually these bacteria hitched a ride with us and all other animals and made a deal. In exchange for a comfortable, safe home inside our colons—an oxygen-free environment if there ever was one (think where the sun don't shine to continue the vampire analogy with a bad pun)—and a steady supply of nutritious foods, they would provide us with a whole roster of health- and longevity-promoting benefits. Our relationship with these microbes was built on symbiosis.

In the ten short years since microbiome research has come into the fore—a mere millisecond in the scientific world—we have discovered a plethora of activities that are mediated by the gut microbiome. It would take volumes to explain each one, so let's focus our attention here on the handful of functions that most impact your energy level and overall well-being.

As you probably would guess given their location, your gut buddies play an important role in your digestion. One important contribution they make is to break down foods that your digestive system can't handle on its own, including the fibers from certain plants. Incredibly, only microbes can digest the rigid outer cell wall of plants contained in raw leaves and vegetables; your digestive enzymes can't accomplish this seemingly simple feat. (As I love to share, even a termite can't digest wood; it needs its own microbiome to do that!) Your hardworking gut buddies also help extract precious energy from food as well as help us extract and manufacture vitamins including K_2, folate, and B_{12}. Their activities also lower your intestinal pH, thereby increasing the solubility and absorption of essential minerals, such as calcium, iron, and magnesium.

In addition to all of this impressive digestive work, your microbes also regulate and provide substrates (building materials) for hormone production, metabolizing amino acids like tryptophan, which you absorb from your diet, to create a substance that is the precursor to the hormone serotonin, a neurotransmitter that helps to regulate mood and feelings of well-being. What's more, your gut buddies may help to break down environmental pollutants and pharmaceuticals, but sadly they are being overwhelmed in that job with the sheer number of chemicals we knowingly and unknowingly ingest.[4] And as a final friendly touch, when your gut wall sloughs off its older cells, they help to reclaim protein from them for your body to use a second time around to build tissues—the ultimate in efficiency!

This is a mere drop in the bucket; but of all the jobs these guys do, one of the most impressive and important is the manufacturing of digestive by-products called postbiotics, which are used to communicate information across bodily systems. Postbiotics are your microbiome's version of text messages, and the emerging research on these gut-derived signaling compounds is quite staggering. Postbiotics influence your hormone levels, your appetite, your mood; your brain structure, function, and development; whether you gain weight or can't lose it; how well you sleep and whether you get anxiety, along with more serious psychological issues—quite literally the gamut of human experience! Though we are only scratching the surface of how our holobiome directs activities throughout our body, we now know that our gut buddies are constantly sharing all sorts of critical data with our cells via the compounds they make, including postbiotics, even giving instructions to your energy-producing mitochondria.

Significantly, your gut buddies also influence the expression of the DNA in your cells. As we now know from the emerging science of epigenetics, our genetic code is not our destiny. In fact, our genes are greatly affected by their environment, which means that we all hold some power over whether our health-giving or disease-giving genes get switched on. Microbiome-produced messages control much of this genetic expression—and the sheer volume of messages they send boggles the mind. Just to make your head spin, one of my colleagues in microbiome research recently shared that they use a supercomputer at his company, Gusto Global, to track the activity of microbes in stool samples. When it comes to detecting which microbes are creating which signals—and which genes get switched on and off as a result—you need ultra-high-level mathematics and exceptional processing power. The complexity of the endeavor rivals outer space exploration.[5]

We are still in the early days of "cracking the code" on the unseen data sharing originating from our biome to our genes, but we do know that when damage to the biome occurs, processing capability is lost, signals get scrambled, and essential compounds are not made—the starting point for fatigue, disease, and aging. And the starting point for this insidious damage takes us back to the very sites where fuel is absorbed and where energy can often be lost—your roots and soil.

Getting Back to Your Roots

Keesha came to her first appointment with me wondering how she could be so pooped. After all, she was a devout vegan who paid a lot of attention to her diet. No boxed or canned goods for her! She cooked daily from scratch. Yet here she was in her twenties, looking and feeling in her fifties, thinner than she wanted to be and plagued by dull skin and dry hair. Her blood tests revealed inflammation, leaky gut, and low thyroid function. No wonder she was exhausted! Keesha's gut, like that of most people today, was on fire.

As you may remember from the last chapter, one of the key drivers of systemic inflammation in the body is a leaky gut. Given how much of an energy drain inflammation creates, a huge focus of the Energy Paradox Program is repairing and healing the gut wall. Now, that doesn't mean that nothing can get through—you'd starve if that were the case. It means that you shore up vulnerabilities so that you are well-protected against mischief makers. A strong gut wall allows authorized material—food molecules, microbial signals, and water—across its border and into your circulatory system, but keeps out unwanted material that could launch your immune system into attack mode. In other words, it lets *in* nutrients that your cells will use as fuel (as well as for growing, repairing, and building tissues), while keeping *out* anything that triggers inflammation and fatigue. It's an entry point and a protective barrier at once, the ultimate customs checkpoint, if you will, where all incoming agents are assessed before they cross over the border.

Here's where the "roots" come in. The inner wall of the intestinal tract has an unusual surface, not flat and smooth like the lining of your arteries. Its surface is shaped into little fingerlike projections (technically called *villi*) that themselves are covered in superfine filaments—your microvilli—which protrude into the dark "soil-filled" cavity of your gut (remember, soil in this context is the content of the gut—food transiting through plus the abundance of microbes residing there) and act to significantly increase its primary absorptive area. Your microvilli are most pronounced in the first twenty feet of small intestine where the majority of food absorption occurs. Picture them as innumerable strands of 1970s shag carpet projecting off the gut wall. In the last five or so feet of the tract—the large intestine, also known as the colon, where less food absorption but lots of water absorption occurs—the projections become less pronounced, closer to a pile carpet. In a sense, you have a twenty-five-foot-long root system, which has roughly the surface area of an *entire tennis court.*

At the bottom of each "root," or villi, is a small crypt that holds something very special—intestinal stem cells that help proliferate new gut lining cells as needed, along with a small deposit of helpful microbes. Why is this so noteworthy? Well, the tissue of your gut lining has a very fast turnover—your entire gut lining regenerates itself on a weekly basis—and when a cell dies and needs to be replaced, a stem cell from the crypt literally divides itself from the others and "crawls" up the microvilli. Your gut wall is designed to regenerate and flourish. These stem cells are exquisitely sensitive to vitamin D, which stimulates them to actively transform to become a gut wall cell. I'm always amazed by how adequate amounts of vitamin D_3 (the form of D your body produces from sunlight on the skin, also available from some animal-sourced foods, and in supplement form) has an almost superpower to reverse fatigue[6]; it certainly does wonders for my autoimmune patients, who are *always* deficient in this vitamin when they first come to see me. Hmm, autoimmune improvement, general fatigue improvement—could this be because vitamin D_3 helps a leaky gut to heal, thus calming the inflammatory war? I believe so, and have shown in my research that is likely the case. Adequate vitamin D_3 supplementation is thus a key component of the Energy Paradox Program.

Halt! Who Goes There?

Now let's zoom in one magnification level further. The entire surface of these microvilli "roots" is covered in a single layer of *enterocytes*—cells that make up the gut lining through which food molecules are absorbed into your circulatory systems. Because your gut wall is only one cell thick, each enterocyte is bonded to its neighbor with a structure called a tight junction that literally "locks" them together so that nothing untoward—say, a pathogen, a noxious chemical you've ingested, a large protein, or a microbiome resident that's gone rogue—sneaks its way between them without permission. If the junctions do begin to weaken and the wall becomes permeable, watch out! The foreign substance gets a nasty surprise: Immune cells interspersed throughout the lining (they actually create a layer of tissue just slightly below the surface level) leap into action. This is the aforementioned and impressive "70 percent" of your immune system that resides in your intestines. It includes T cells and Tregs, natural killer cells, macrophages, and B cells, many of which are installed with the scanner-like TLRs you met in the last chapter. Remember how I said they take their job seriously? Sensing an outsider elbowing its way through your gut wall, they will very quickly sound the alarms.

Let's revisit the second "L" of inflammation, lectins, to discover why even a healthy-seeming whole-foods diet can contribute to leaky gut and an overactive immune response—and why making the right diet and lifestyle choices for your gut buddies has such an impact. Lectins—the sticky proteins in most grains, legumes and beans, and some fruit and vegetable peels and seeds—have an uncanny ability to trigger production of a protein called *zonulin* in the gut wall cells. Zonulin, in turn, activates a switch that breaks apart the tight junctions, creating leaky gut. This "opens the doors" for unwanted matter like lectins, and even living bacteria, to slip across the border and generate inflammation. Now, lectins can only do this if they've made it through four layers of defense: mouth saliva and mucus, stomach acid, the gut buddies in the microbiome that have a knack for breaking them down and eating them, and the intestinal mucus lining the gut wall that should bind them up nicely, so they can't cause zonulin to activate. The denser your mucus is the better your body can contain and trap the lectins in your diet—which is why those with terrific gut health may not have big issues consuming them.

Dense, sticky mucus provides a further benefit; in addition to keeping zonulin from being triggered, it invites the gut bugs that produce *anti-inflammatory* by-products (postbiotics) to cozy on up nice and close to the wall, contributing to a calmer and less inflamed gut environment. What helps the gut cells secrete ample mucus? The presence of a certain kind of gut buddy called *Akkermansia muciniphila*. Think of the gut's mucosal lining as part of a very sophisticated firewall system. In a perfect example of "roots and soil" symbiosis, a healthy, thriving gut ecology helps you to make more of this mucus that in turn helps your roots and soil coexist and stay strong.

Unfortunately, today's diet replete with whole grains and other lectin-containing foods (which have no longer been properly prepared to render them less harmful) forces this protective mucus to work overtime, desperately working to bind up the lectins. When mucus production can't keep up with the demand from the diet, it gets thin and scanty, leaving the gut wall vulnerable, which contributes to broken tight junctions and more inflammation. Add to that the smorgasbord of chemicals that most modern humans ingest, from pesticides to over-the-counter NSAIDs (nonsteroidal anti-inflammatory drugs, like ibuprofen), which also destroy the gut wall, and many of us have mastered the recipe for leaky gut.

If you're like Keesha and many of my other savvy patients, you might balk at the idea that traditional foods like bulgur, oats, and beans could be contributing to leaky gut and, ergo, the fatigue of inflammation. As I told Keesha, unfair as it may be, the intact defense systems that protected her ancestors from zonulin-triggering lectins have been weakened by constant assaults from our modern diet and lifestyle. But there is a way back to what has been lost. After going lectin-free and repairing her gut wall and microbiome, as you will learn how to do in Part II, Keesha experienced a great turnaround. Within months her energy returned with a vengeance, she achieved a healthy body weight as her intestinal absorption improved, and despite the fact that she had to give up a few of her favorite foods, she shared a sentiment I've heard from many patients: "Feeling well never tasted so good!"

Now, if you're wondering what all this talk about your endlessly chattering microbes and mucus-covered roots has to do with our epidemic of exhaustion and inflammation, the answer is: a lot.

Your Gut Buddies and Your Immune System: Allies at the Front Line

The diversity of your microbial ecosystem plays a significant role in your immune health. A diverse and dynamic gut biome contains multiple strains of bacteria that literally teach the immune system to not only tolerate the microbial "foreigners" living near the gut wall, but also to trust the signals and messages they send about how things are going in the outside world. (Remember, they are your cloud computer sending real-time data about changes and possible dangers in your environment.) By contrast, if the balance in your biome tips toward less salubrious strains due to your diet, lifestyle, and stress, then this communication is drowned out. The TLRs on the white blood cells and macrophages sense the presence of these more mischievous microbes and—bingo—an inflammation-inducing battle begins. If your mucus lining is scanty and your gut is already permeable, you have a double whammy: Your immune cells detect foreign invaders, send soldiers to the wall, and in the process of trying to kill the invaders, they kill your own cells alongside. This makes for a weaker and even *more* permeable gut, which means *more* of the inflammatory microbial particles (LPSs), and even live bacteria and fungi, can reach distant organs through circulation, inciting inflammation around your whole body. These escaping microbes make it to your fat tissue (inflaming it, which makes you gain more fat), your liver and heart (contributing to issues like fatty liver and cardiomyopathies), and even your brain (creating cognitive impairment). It is truly remarkable how a simple change in gut bacteria can take you from a place of peace and quiet and abundant energy to a full-blown, and fully exhausting, forest fire!

Not surprisingly because they live "cheek to cheek," your gut buddies exist in a kind of constant dance with your immune system.[7] The gut buddies teach the immune cells how to respond when confronted by a foreign substance or even the microbes themselves. (In technical terms, this is known as dictating the "tone" of the immune response.) In return, the immune system helps promote a stable microbiome by fostering diversity and literally selecting which bugs it wants to tolerate and which it doesn't, even though all of those microbes with foreign DNA are not a part of "you."[8] This dance has been in motion since you were born, and even before, since you were in utero. Your microbiome has actually contributed to the very *development* of your immune cells. Even as a fetus, your microbiome was instructing your developing immune system. And for those of you who made your entrance into the world through your mother's birth canal and received her breast milk, your mother's microbes helped to fine-tune the way your immune cells respond to potential threats, from tree pollen to peanuts to viruses. Your microbiome shows your immune system the ropes as it matures, so it doesn't fire off at every little squabble and learns to keep its cool.

If the dots are connecting, a couple of "aha"s might be hitting you at this moment: Yes, this is why mothers are encouraged to breastfeed their infants (breast milk is loaded with bacteria and fungi, plus it brims with the exact types of sugars a baby's gut buddies feast on to flourish and grow). And this is why small children, until recently, were not discouraged from playing in the dirt and picking snacks up off the floor—the first three years of life are a time for monumental gut–immune system education, and the more inputs from nature the better. Over time the learning continues little by little until a massive immune system archive exists of what's "good" and "bad."

This education and archive-building is the ideal scenario. Your diverse, flourishing biome wants to be in constant communication with your immune system and your mitochondria, a cross talk that is known as *trans-kingdom communication* (very Star Wars–like, eh?). Except that our signals are often scrambled today. Due to a combination of microbiome disruption and damage to the gut wall—and changes in the way we enter the world and spend early childhood—these messages are not always being sent or received as they should. Miscommunication is occurring! With a microbiome that's less capable of making anti-inflammatory signals, your immune system receives too many messages to "attack" and not nearly enough messages to "stand down" (one unfortunate example of this poor communication is the recent, dramatic rise in allergies to peanuts and bee stings). What's worse, and as we will soon discuss, your confused immune system can start to attack the very thing it needs for energy production: your mitochondria! How could that be? Well, remember that your mitochondria are ancient bacteria. A hyper-activated immune system attacks bacteria if they encounter them, without first asking for ID.

Pruned Roots: A Sure Path to Exhaustion

When your gut wall is constantly inflamed, it becomes so damaged that the roots get pruned. That's less of a metaphor than it sounds. When inflammation runs amok, the villi that project off the gut wall can become stunted. This drastically reduces the surface area available in your intestines for absorbing proteins, sugars, fatty acids, and minerals and vitamins—all the things that feed into your energy production system. Now, your body is smart; it will steal protein from your muscles to feed this need. But when this becomes your norm, it eats away at your muscle tissue, causing muscle wasting—not the kind of "skinny" you want. This combination of muscle wasting and being totally worn out is quite typical of those with celiac disease and inflammatory bowel diseases like Crohn's disease, and it's all from damage to the primary absorptive surface of the gut.

If your fatigue is compounded by symptoms like muscle-mass loss or unexplained weight loss, it's important to see a doctor, as you may have a serious intestinal disorder. The good news is that over the last two decades, I've treated many patients with these issues using my Paradox programs, and I'm happy to say that 94 percent of them have recovered. Their roots heal, they begin absorbing nutrients, muscles are spared, and energy returns. What a testament to the body's ability to fix itself, Hippocrates' *veriditas* in action. So if you are a senior who has been told that your proteins are low or that your muscles are wasting—or even a younger person who is losing weight and told to eat more protein—I have news for you: You don't need more protein, you need to grow some new roots and stop damaging the ones you have!

The Fiber Paradox

Our five pounds of probiotic bacteria need to eat, just like we do—and their favorite things to eat are *prebiotic* foods. Your gut buddies "compost" these foods for you, and in the process, create special kinds of fatty acids and, we are now discovering, generate gases that communicate information from your microbiome to your cells (and the mitochondria within them). While you would've had to have lived under a rock not to know about probiotics in this day and age, it's actually the other two "Ps" that should get the limelight, because the probiotics in and of themselves aren't doing much for you if they aren't getting fed the prebiotics they need to make these extraordinarily significant compounds.

So, what's the best source of these important prebiotic foods that fuel the production of postbiotics? In a word: fiber. I've found that this nutrient is hugely underappreciated in the American diet—most of my patients have no idea how much fiber they consume in a day. Heck, many of them don't even know what foods contain fiber! (If you do, congratulations, but trust me, most people do not.)

The term "fiber" refers to a variety of complex carbohydrates, including resistant starches and other nondigestible sugars that "resist" being broken down in the small intestine. While the small intestine has the enzymes to digest *simple* starches (which are made up of lots of sugar molecules strung together in a chain), it lacks the enzymes to break apart resistant starches' *complex*, tightly bound sugar molecules or intact cell walls or both; thus this fiber passes through relatively unscathed. When you eat "undigestible" carbohydrates, you typically eat them alongside digestible proteins, fats, and simple sugars in your meal. The undigestible mix of plant fibers from your salad, sauerkraut, or asparagus slows transit of these other foods, keeping the absorption of simple sugars gradual and steady so that your body, and more important, your energy-producing mitochondria, can assimilate the nutrients in a slow and steady fashion. Eventually, as components from digested food cross into your bloodstream to provide energy to your cells, the remaining fiber continues on down to the large intestine, and a certain subset of it known as *soluble fiber* meets its maker—your microbiome.

Now, here's a bit of a shocking statistic. The diets of our hunter-gatherer ancestors consisted of about 150 grams of fiber *per day* (the Hadzas have a similar fiber intake today). The average modern American diet contains about 20 to 25 grams of fiber.[9] (Even with a pretty high vegetable and plant intake, it tends to max out at 60 grams.) And if you are doing a keto diet, you may consume almost no fiber. We live in an age of fiber deficit, and the less fiber we eat, the sicker we get[10]—and vice versa. When your gut buddies aren't fed the foods they need to make anti-inflammatory, energy-producing signaling molecules (postbiotics), rampant inflammation and exhaustion is likely to take hold. And when you're dog-tired at the end of the day, it's a lot more tempting to reach for a bag of chips than to get up off the couch and make yourself a salad.

"Okay, doc, I got it," you may be thinking. "I'll eat more fiber! I'll buy some high-fiber cereal or bake a batch of bran muffins and get this issue squared away." Well, while I'm glad you're willing to support your gut buddies and make some changes to your diet, I'm afraid those changes are exactly the wrong ones to make.

When you eat a bowl of bran-fiber cereal or a bran muffin, you are not in fact feeding your biome in the way I've described, and therefore not getting the health benefits you likely assume. The fact that a whole generation of people were raised on the idea of sitting down to a breakfast full of whole-grain "goodness" has been built on a fundamental misunderstanding (lie?) about the way fiber works. It's a long story, but suffice to say that the pioneering fiber scientists overemphasized the importance of *whole grain* fibers, unaware of their negative (lectin-filled) impact. A grain-based food system ran with this concept, and voila: a long-standing misconception that launched a massively profitable industry of multigrain breads, bran-filled cereals, fiber bars, and the like.

Meanwhile, in the last twenty-five years, huge gains have been made in the field of fiber science. We now know that a balanced and energy-promoting fiber-rich diet is one full of soluble and *insoluble fibers* from plant leaves, stems, tubers, and roots, rather than the hulls of grains. These are the fibers that reach the bugs in your gut microbiome and are eaten by *them*, not you. Since there are quite a few types of fiber, let's simplify the subject so it feels doable to add prebiotics to your diet—like a good gardener, I want you to feel comfortable working with a combo of mulches for your soil.

We can broadly divide the fiber category into two groups: soluble fiber (meaning that it dissolves in water) and insoluble fiber (which is insoluble in water—think wheat bran). Soluble fiber can be fermented by your gut buddies to make energy that allows them to multiply and produce postbiotics. Some insoluble fiber, like cellulose, can be also eaten by the gut buddies, which is why achieving a vegetable-filled diet is such an important health- and energy-boosting goal, because most plant foods contain both types of fiber in various proportions. But other types of insoluble fiber, like wheat bran, act as a sharp irritant to the gut wall.[11] No wonder it makes you move your bowels!

When it comes to soluble fibers, you may already know that some fruits are good sources, like crispy pears (crispy, not overripe, to keep the fructose content low) and avocados. However, certain soluble fibers deliver the *most* bang for fermenting buck—they're the ones our gut buddies really love: inulin, oligofructose, and fructooligosaccharides (FOSs), and the rest of the fructans. You can find these fibers in Jerusalem artichokes, chicory root, onions, leeks, garlic, green bananas, dandelion roots, and asparagus. Inulin is one of the best-studied prebiotic fibers, shown to be present in thousands of types of plants—like chicory root and the chicory family of vegetables, many of which would have been part of your ancestors' hunter-gatherer buffet! In fact, researchers studying dry cave deposits in northern Mexico have estimated that as much as 135 grams of early humans' fiber intake came from inulin in the form of desert plants![12] Sounds like an absolute feast for their gut buddies. Yet in today's diet, inulin accounts for only a few grams per day of your fiber intake—if that.

In a neighboring fiber category to inulin are the resistant starches, which are found in foods you might already be familiar with, like millet, parsnips, turnips, sweet potatoes and yams, green papaya and rutabaga, as well as green plantains, cassava, jicama, taro root, and tiger nuts. (Fun fact: Cooked starches when chilled and then reheated contain more-resistant starch than when eaten fresh out of the oven or stove.) Resistant starches, as you'll remember, partially "resist" the digestive enzymes in your small intestine and make their way into your colon relatively intact. Given that it's an oxygen-free environment in there, resistant starches are broken down via fermentation. You beer and wine fans out there may know that fermentation is an anaerobic (without oxygen) process called *glycolysis* that uses sugars or amino acids to generate ATP. The same thing happens in your gut when you eat resistant starches—when your probiotic bacteria ferment the starches, energy is generated, giving them the fuel to replicate, which adds to their diversity and abundance so that they, in turn, can produce more postbiotics.

When you eat a low-fiber diet—one full of highly refined carbohydrates stripped of naturally occurring fibers, or a diet that contains far more fat and protein than plant matter—most of the absorption of sugars, fats, and proteins happens way upstream, at the top of your small intestine. That's a problem for three important reasons:

First, these foods are absorbed almost immediately in your small intestine—your body doesn't have to do any real work to digest them. What this means is that you don't burn nearly as many calories in the process of digestion as you do with fiber-rich foods, which require energy to be broken down[13] (the geeky name for the energy used in digestion is *postprandial thermogenic responses*). And by losing the benefit of burning calories as you digest, your net gain of calories increases, and so does your waistline and weight. Think of it this way: The more processed your food is, the less "work" is done to break it into absorbable pieces, and the more net calories you absorb. Ouch.

Second, this meal of refined food contributes to an energy "rush hour" in which your energy factories, the mitochondria, get hit by too many sugars, fats, and proteins all at once. This overwhelms the mitochondria's ability to handle fuel sources efficiently and safely and, though it is rarely discussed, it is at the core of modern mitochondrial dysfunction and a key driver of fatigue and insulin resistance. You will learn a lot more about this in the next chapter.

Last, as you've probably deduced, a diet stripped of fiber deprives the gut buddies downstream in your colon—your soil's superorganisms, with their incredible processing power—of the raw materials they need to do the important work of guiding the ship. This seemingly small point actually has tremendous consequences. As processed foods and fast foods have increasingly replaced whole foods across the Western world, our gut microbes are going hungry. In fact, new research suggests that the sensations of hunger we experience may actually originate from our microbes sending the message to our brain that they need to be fed! We are literally starving the vital "virtual organ" we need to support our health, and we are paying the price with chronic disease and chronically low energy levels.[14]

When you're eating the right amount of fiber, you'll know it—there will be striking evidence. My good friend and colleague Dr. Terry Wahls, who reversed her MS by following an integrative protocol that includes eating nine cups of vegetables a day, describes the huge amount of output coming out downstream that is common when you eat plenty of fiber. That volume comes from the copious amounts of bacteria growing in your intestines that have feasted on the fibers' sugars. If you've transitioned to a plant-rich, high-fiber diet you've likely experienced this proof yourself—you might have been surprised by your suddenly much larger bowel movements. Far from something to be alarmed about, however, this is a sign that your gut buddies have been well fed, have replicated in number, and in the process, have made powerful postbiotic compounds for your body—and now that their work is done, this generation of buddies is moving out.

If the visual alone doesn't sway you, chew on this: For every pound of these fibers you eat, you make a third of a pound of new bacteria. Meaning, if you eat the right foods, a third of the potential calories you swallow is used to feed them instead of you. It's like you get to eat 30 percent more food without gaining an ounce! More important, in exchange for feeding them, you will experience a huge improvement in intestinal health and overall energy levels because many of the postbiotic compounds they produce will help heal the gut and boost mitochondrial health. That's right, they help a leaky gut wall to proliferate strong new cells, which reduces inflammation, which reduces fatigue . . . all from proper feeding of your gut buddies.[15] One last thought before moving on. Do you know the most common complaint of an Atkins, keto, or carnivore diet? If you guessed constipation, you are right: no "food" to feed the gut buddies, no new little gut buddy babies. On my plan you'll be happy to know that two of the benefits are prodigious bowel movements plus more energy! Now that will put a spring into your step!

So what actually occurs when you do feed your gut buddies what they long for, and create a home that allows them to thrive? They do that all-important work of generating "text messages" that signal all sorts of activities in your body to switch on and off. These postbiotic messages take many forms (infinitely more, I believe, than we currently know). For the purposes of keeping things (relatively) simple, we'll break them into the two categories known to have the most effects on your energy and well-being: the well-studied short-chain fatty acids and the newly discovered gasotransmitters (also called *gasomessengers*).

Short-Chain Fatty Acids: The Healing and Energizing SCFAs

Short-chain fatty acids, or SCFAs, are the real superstars of postbiotics. Your gut buddies produce three short-chain fatty acids, but the most important one when it comes to energy production is butyrate, which contributes about 10 percent to your system-wide energy production. It's especially critical to energy production in the gut; in fact, your colon cells use butyrate as their primary fuel source.[16,17] They literally live on this stuff!

Furthermore, in the "cheek to cheek" dance between your biome and your immune system, *butyrate* is a key signaler driving anti-inflammatory hormone production. This fatty acid's pacifying messages also communicate directly to intestinal macrophages, ensuring they don't mistake friendly bacteria in the gut for enemies.[18] To put a bow on it, butyrate also helps regulate cell growth and differentiation, which helps prevent colon cells from becoming cancerous.[19] Moreover, lack of adequate SCFAs has been shown to play a significant role in the development of obesity and metabolic syndrome, as well as bowel disease (like colitis and Crohn's) and certain types of cancer.[20,21]

It doesn't stop there. The butyrate that isn't used in the gut moves into your lymphatic system and bloodstream, circulating to all your cells, where it attaches to cellular membranes in order to deliver information. Butyrate then journeys even deeper inside the cells, to the mitochondrial membrane, where they deliver the message to your energy workers that conditions down in the engine room are all good, hence, "Keep producing energy!" This postbiotic cross talk (as it's officially dubbed) can also instruct your genes, and gives real-time updates to systems across your body. Your body is so well engineered that if it *doesn't* get those reaffirming postbiotic messages, it senses something may be wrong—and until the cause is figured out, it'll throttle back on energy production as a precautionary measure. It's kind of like seeing a fault light come up indicating issues with your car's fuel line. Instead of pressing the pedal to the metal, you're going to slow down and conserve any gas you have.

Step on the Gas for More Energy

Here's a paradox you probably weren't expecting to find in this book: Belly-made gases are good for your health. For most of your life you've likely gone to great lengths to try to avoid gas or have been red-faced at its presence. Perhaps you've even suffered at times with a painful buildup of gas, a common symptom of conditions like irritable bowel syndrome (IBS) and small intestinal bacterial overgrowth (SIBO). But the bad rap intestinal gases have gotten in our culture is not fully deserved. When produced in the right amounts, new research shows that postbiotic gases play several important roles in the body, including acting as a second set of powerful signaling agents, similar to short-chain fatty acids. In this way, postbiotic gases invisibly influence infinite amounts of your bodily functions including your inflammation levels, brain clarity, and mitochondrial energy production. And though they're considered rude to discuss in polite company, the gasotransmitters are possibly even more critical to your energy than the short-chain fatty acids. So, let's air this out, shall we?

The most abundant intestinal gases in the human body are nitrogen and carbon dioxide. They primarily originate from inhaled air that you swallowed, so most of us who suffer from "gas and bloating" are actually air swallowers from talking and breathing. However, some gases are produced by bacterial fermentation, like hydrogen, methane, and hydrogen sulfide, as well as the aforementioned CO_2. These have only very recently joined the league of gasotransmitters led by nitric oxide—the first gasotransmitter "discovered" to be not just a vasodilator but also a signaling molecule used by the microbiome to influence a wide array of bodily functions.[22] This breakthrough discovery garnered a Nobel Prize in 1998.[23] Who ever thought that your gas could be worthy of a Nobel Prize?!

Okay, so you make some gas, you pass an embarrassing fart that smells like rotten eggs (that's hydrogen sulfide), you play the old Boy Scout trick of lighting it with a BIC lighter (that's hydrogen gas, think *Hindenburg*, highly flammable), or you contribute to greenhouse gases like the cows (that's methane gas). No big deal, you might think, that's just the cost of doing digestion. Except these biome-generated gases, which it turns out are *all* constantly sending signals to the cells in your body, are a *really* big deal. For example, not only did nitric oxide signaling function get recognized with a Nobel, it actually got an even bigger accolade in 2019, when researchers declared it to be a hitherto unrecognized sophisticated system that "communicates with and controls the host's DNA *like a chemical language* instead of single words."[24] How's that for impressive? And methane, which has possibly the worst rap of all gases for its negative effects on climate, is both crucial for proper mitochondrial function and an important modulator of inflammation.[25] The gasotransmitters produced in your gut play an incredibly important role in your inner ecosystem as they serve as the primary language of "trans-kingdom" or interspecies communication: in other words, the "cross talk" or "operating system" between the bacteria in your microbiome and your body's cells.

Gas Overload

There's no denying that conditions like IBS and SIBO include significant discomfort caused by an overproduction of gas building up in the intestines And anytime you feel chronically bloated and achy, you're going to lose your get-up-and-go. For that reason, there's been a kind of "anti-gas vendetta," in which entire movements and books are devoted to eliminating from the diet any fermentable sugar to relieve the discomfort (such as the famous GAPS diet and SCD, or specific carbohydrate diet, to name two). There are even suggestions that gluten intolerance symptoms aren't caused by the gluten family of proteins opening the tight junctions of the gut and triggering inflammation, but rather by the FODMAPs in grains (FODMAPs stands for fermentable oligo-, di-, mono-saccharides, and polyols).

Many of my patients had been on or are currently on one of these diets when they first see me, and some have had symptomatic improvement with these programs. While yes, fermentation of various sugars by bacteria—but more likely yeasts like candida—do produce gases, and some gases will distend the intestines and cause bloating and/or pain and cramping, it's no reason to eliminate all gas-producing foods from your diet. What the Energy Paradox Program will do is give your gut buddies the right amount of the right fibers to produce just the right amount of these all-important gasotransmitters, without overdoing it.

Gasotransmitters are intended to exist in a "sweet spot": neither too much, nor too little, but to quote Goldilocks, "just right." (In non–fairy tale language, that's called following a hormetic curve; you'll learn more about hormesis in Chapter 6). During my years of working with patients, I have almost always found that when a patient follows my Paradox program, even if they arrived with the diagnoses of IBS, SIBO, candida, and the resulting chronic fatigue that can come with them, the conditions resolve once we address their diet and give the microbiome the right foods and fibers.

When it comes to your energy equation, there are three gaso-transmitters generated by your gut bugs that are most important. First up is hydrogen. The smallest molecule in the universe, it can rapidly pass through the intestinal wall and diffuse into your cells where it counters damaging molecules known as oxidants. We now know that hydrogen is produced by many gut microbes, and over the last decade we've discovered that it is both a powerful antioxidant and signaling molecule. Though an over-buildup of hydrogen gas may cause you to wince, when hitting the sweet spot, it activates the Nrf2-Keap1 pathway, which regulates hundreds of protective proteins and enzymes involved in the crucial cellular protection known as antioxidation and the equally important pro-cesses of detoxification. Moreover, hydrogen can literally "turn down" inflammation by downregulating another pathway. Less inflammation equals less wasted energy equals more energy for you! See, I told you gas deserved more respect.

Hydrogen gas can also be used as a therapeutic agent, particularly when administered in drinking water. If you've heard of the new trend of "hydrogen water" or listened to my podcast about it—or if you've seen it and wondered if it is just a new way to sell expen-sive H_2O—I can tell you that it is most certainly not a gimmick. Hydrogen-dissolved water has been shown to reduce the damaging stress that occurs inside your cells (called *oxidative stress*) via the removal of reactive oxygen species (you'll learn more about these shortly), with knock-on effects such as reducing the symptoms of obesity, metabolic syndrome, and Parkinson's disease.[26] The fact that patients with Parkinson's disease have a dramatically lower abundance of hydrogen-producing bacteria in their microbiome suggests that the hydrogen produced in the gut may have an impact on the prevention of this horrible neurodegenerative disease.[27,28] Wait a minute, read that again: Parkinson's patients have less hydrogen-producing bacteria species than is normal. Were their brain cells deprived of the signaling data they need to do their jobs right? Or were they deprived of the protective antioxidants they need to thrive, or both? The evidence points to both. Time for a real "gut check," right? In fact, over 1,500 studies have shown that hydrogen alleviates illness and improves outcomes in a wide range of pathological conditions.[29]

After hydrogen is produced by one set of gut buddies, another set of microbes transforms hydrogen into additional gases, like hydrogen sulfide and methane, in a process called *cross-feeding*. In this case, sulfur (partially sourced from cruciferous vegetables) is cross-fed with hydrogen to make more gaseous messengers. This is a perfect example of ecosystem interdependence: The different strains of bacteria in your gut feed off of each other's leftovers, and in so doing, are able to then contribute to the health of the whole ecosystem, including you.

Hydrogen sulfide is not something you'd normally think you'd want to cheer—after all, this "rotten egg" smelling gas has long been known to be highly toxic. Back when it was first identified in the seventeenth century by a German scientist, it was believed that this gas emanated from sewer systems, and was to blame for a painful inflammatory eye disease in sewer workers. While a large buildup of hydrogen sulfide in the tissues absolutely *is* toxic and damaging, including to your mitochondria and their energy production, what we didn't know was that in the right amounts, it is not only *not* toxic, it's absolutely critical to the functioning of your cells.[30] Moreover, we now know it helps to maintain the gut mucus layer integrity, helping to prevent leaky gut.

Hydrogen sulfide is also a neurotransmitter and neuromodulator that can help your brain learn and retain memories better while offering further protection from neurodegenerative diseases. (In fact, all of the principle gasotransmitters facilitate communication between neurons so that your brain function stays sharp.)[31] In addition to its brain-boosting powers, hydrogen sulfide appears to play a significant role in cardiovascular health, protecting against high cholesterol and high blood pressure.[32] Interestingly, however, you can undo this protective benefit with the wrong diet. Eating a high-fat diet has been shown to decrease hydrogen sulfide metabolization and actually promote atherosclerotic heart disease.[33,34] And remember what I said earlier about stiff blood vessels and no energy? The same applies to your heart's energy production. Think about that: A high-fat diet can cause heart disease, not because the *fat* is inherently bad for you, but because your gut buddies didn't have the right nutrients to make enough hydrogen sulfide to protect your blood vessels. Paging your cardiologist! Stop the statins and prescribe broccoli?[35] Hydrogen sulfide is so important that it is not only made in the gut, it's also created within cells where it plays a role in the mitochondrial energy chain; it can actually act as an energy substrate for mitochondria when times are tough. And if your energy is low, I assure you times are tough for your mitochondria!

Unfortunately, the converse is true—and it is an almost completely unknown driver of everyday fatigue. If your body senses the absence of these essential gases, due to a microbiome that is underfed or unsupported, it can go into energy-saving mode: *Better slow down operations; something is up.*[36,37,38]

You can probably start to picture why those folks still hunting and gathering off the land—like the Hadzas, who seemingly are able to get more energy from the same amount of caloric intake as sedentary office workers—are able to pull this off. Their gut biome is well fed and producing copious postbiotics, helping to ensure that any inflammation is tamed and under control, and—as you'll see shortly—their gut buddies are working *for* their energy production system by sending energy substrates when needed, especially when it's a long time between hunted and gathered meals! (New bumper sticker: *It's the fiber, stupid!*) While it might seem intimidating to hear that your gut is where so much of the action starts when it comes to feeling energized, clear, and focused, it's actually encouraging. Studies show that when you take out what harms the gut wall and gut buddies, and add in what's needed, you have the power to rapidly change and alter your microbiome,[39] creating positive shifts within days.

The universe of bacteria in your body controls much of your health; and you, mere human, have a *lot* of control over how well they do their jobs because the vast majority of this communication is dependent on your daily choices. These include the foods you eat, the chemicals you encounter daily or not, and even the way you time your meals (more on this in Chapter 6). It all begins with your attentiveness to your roots and soil. Are you trying to cultivate a vital, robust organism with deadened dirt, a dearth of compost, and a steady stream of synthetic chemicals? Many of us are practically like walking plants in an overfarmed, monocropped field; boosted by crutches, weak on the inside and with an inner ecosystem that is under constant attack. Thankfully for you, that's about to change for the better. But before you learn how to do that, we need to turn to the second "M" of the energy equation: your mitochondria.

ENERGY MYTH #3: Doc, I've Got Adrenal Fatigue!

There's a lot of confusion out there when it comes to the interplay of stress, adrenal function, and fatigue. My practice is inundated with tired, brain foggy, and overall poorly functioning patients who have been told (either by a well-meaning practitioner or by Dr. Google) that they have "adrenal fatigue." Others come in with what they have self-diagnosed as "high cortisol levels," and attribute this to their stubborn weight gain or poor sleep. Frequently, my type A patients (perfectionists that they are) blame themselves for getting into what they think is an adrenal/cortisol mess. "I burned out my adrenals working too hard, drinking too much caffeine, not going to yoga," they may say, likely inspired by internet myths. Others have spent a small fortune on supplements to try to "fix" those darned broken adrenals.

If adrenal fatigue has been on your tired, poorly functioning mind lately, dear reader, please know that while you are right that chronic stress is throwing things out of balance, it's highly unlikely your adrenals have reached their max and have quit, nor are you flooding your system with an egregious amount of cortisol. Chances are more likely that, like 95 percent of my tired patients, your adrenal glands are just fine. You read that correctly. In fact, of the thousands of patients I've treated, fewer than ten have had an abnormally low morning cortisol level. However, similar to the way your cells can become resistant to insulin when receptors for insulin get blocked by ceramides, your adrenal hormone receptors can also get blocked, making you resistant to receiving the messages these hormones want to give you, and actually contributing to more inflammation—which may be the thing that is making you so tired. Let me explain.

Your adrenal glands produce the hormone cortisol, along with adrenaline and norepinephrine, which are stimulating and glucose-raising hormones. These are some of the things they do to get you going in the morning (perhaps you could call them your get-up-and-go hormones!). They naturally ebb and flow throughout a twenty-four-hour cycle. In most of my patients, even the type As who report being "tired and wired," the actual circulating cortisol level in their bloodstream is within a normal range. (Untreated, chronic elevated cortisol is a real cause for concern, because it can damage your hippocampus, the memory center of your brain, but I just don't see it that often.) Rather, being chronically stressed means you are producing so much norepinephrine, adrenaline, and cortisol that your cell receptors have become less sensitive to them. This in itself is something of a problem: It seems as if prolonged stress causes glucocorticoid receptor resistance (GCR), which then interferes with the hypothalamic-pituitary axis's appropriate regulation of inflammation.[40] When the receptors are messed up, inflammation is never quelled. And boy, are you tired from that!

Your cells have elegant ways of buffering themselves against too much of a "good thing." Just like mitochondria protect themselves from the onslaught of too many calories, particularly sugar, by becoming resistant to them, so too do cells protect themselves from chronic stimulation of adrenal and cortisol hormones by becoming resistant to them. (It's kind of like your teenager's ability to tune out your voice.) Your adrenals are fine, your cells have just stopped listening. Rather than spending your savings on adrenal supplements and tinctures, or beating yourself up about your morning coffee, I'd encourage you to work on the larger project of reducing inflammation and getting on the circadian rhythm–enhancing program that is the "C^2" of the $E = M^2C^2$ equation.

CHAPTER 4

YOUR MIGHTY MITOCHONDRIA ARE ALL MIXED UP

The crux of the twenty-first-century energy crisis comes down to the title of this chapter. If you're feeling the weight of fatigue you just can't shake, I would wager that the scenario I'm about to describe is quietly unfolding inside all your cells. It's a bold assertion, I realize. But the vast majority of people today are inadvertently bombarding their cellular energy system with *too much fuel*. And that is the conundrum at the core of *The Energy Paradox*: You are overfed but simultaneously underpowered. That's because there's a mismatch between the conditions required by your four quadrillion energy workers—otherwise known as your mitochondria—and the nutrition they're getting from you. Deprived of the raw materials they need to create energy, and yet bombarded with literally tons of inferior-grade fuel, they're being forced to take some desperate measures to try to keep energy production on track.

I can assure you that mitochondrial dysfunction is at the root of not only widespread fatigue, but also many of the illnesses that affect millions of people today, including heart disease, cardiomyopathies, diabetes, metabolic syndrome, cancer, obesity, autoimmune conditions, and neurodegenerative diseases.[1] In fact, persistent fatigue is a warning sign that your mitochondria are overtaxed and unsupported, and may be on the brink of staging a strike. For obvious reasons, you don't want your essential workers curtailing efforts or shutting down factory lines, which starves your cells, tissues, and organs of the energy they need to function. On some level, you could say that all disease is a function of an energy deficit. Illness stems from the "dis-ease" of the mighty mitochondria.

Small in Size, Mighty in Number

At the risk of dating myself, I'll admit that I always picture mito-chondria as little clones of Mighty Mouse—the character from the 1950s cartoon that I loved to watch as a kid. He was a mighty but minuscule superhero who really did, as the theme song promised, "come to save the day"—just as your mitochondria do in real life. These tiny rod-shaped organelles reside inside of almost every cell of your body, where they live in great numbers—there can be thousands of them in some cells. They're especially numerous in the cells of the tissues and organs that require a lot of energy, like your muscles, brain, heart, and liver. As diminutive as they may be, they play a vital role in keeping you alive, converting your daily deposits of food—which are broken down into glu-cose from carbohydrates, amino acids from proteins, and fatty acids from fats—into the energy "currency" your cells can actually spend, ATP.

Chances are you don't often think about this invisible activity. Yet the mitochondria's effort is Herculean. Your body's demands for energy are quite staggering. An average-sized person in good health makes around 140 pounds of ATP every day.[2] You read that right: 140 *pounds*. Since by a fairly conservative estimate, you eat around 3.5 pounds of food per day, that's a tremendous return on investment. And if you're thinking, "I barely weigh 140 pounds, where on earth did all that ATP go?" The answer is: You spent it! (And that's just at rest. During periods of activity, the demands are much higher.) No wonder the health of your mitochondria is so crucial to your get-up-and-go!

In Chapter 3, you read how these powerhouses have a fascinating origin story, evolving from bacteria that became engulfed by the precursors to eukaryotic cells, cells that form the basis of most of life on earth. The transformation of these ancestral bacteria (or proto-mitochondria) into current mitochondria has been fundamental to the evolution of life.[3] Nearly 1.5 billion years ago, these ancient bacteria evolved in a hydrogen sulfide–rich environment—before the oxygen-rich atmosphere was formed—that helped them manufacture energy, an ability they still retain in their new homes within our cells. Besides using hydrogen sulfide, the bacteria helped these early cells to respire, that is, use oxygen to make energy; in return, the cells gave them a home. Over time, the mitochondrion took shape as an essential component of the cell. But it retained many of its ancestral bacterial features; mitochondria not only have a unique double membrane that separates them from the rest of the cell's contents, but, like your gut buddies, they also have their own DNA. This means that they can divide at the same time their host cells divide, but they can also divide at any time *separate from cell division* through a process called *mitogenesis*. The fact that they can replicate on their own, inside their host cell, is critical for your ability to increase your energy production. After all, more energy workers can create more energy.

The reason I'm sharing this ancient history is twofold. First, because your microbiome and mitochondria still exist in a "sisterhood" of sorts, tethered by their shared bacterial past. As with the first colony of microbes that you inherited from your mother's body, you also inherited your mitochondria from your mother. And like good sisters, they communicate often, signaling via postbiotics. Your gut microbes chat constantly with your mitochondria, letting them know if all is well and they should keep making energy, or things are amiss and energy production should slow down.

Second, because your mitochondria are bacterial in nature, they can come under scrutiny from your ever-vigilant immune system. Should things go wrong with your mitochondria, damaged or even dead mitochondria can slip out of their cellular container and into your circulation, where the immune system scans them and may determine them to be a threat. This scenario becomes quite a paradox indeed: Your energy factories may actually contribute to energy-draining inflammation.

The role of mitochondria doesn't stop with making ATP; these guys also influence the very fate of the cells they inhabit since they play a part in regulating cellular homeostasis, including balancing cellular calcium levels (a small-seeming detail that has a massive impact), and driving much of the communication that takes place within cells (a function called *intracellular signaling*). In other words, they tell your cells' DNA and other organelles what to do. They also play key roles in the production of multiple steroid hormones, including the sex hormones, like estrogen and testosterone, and they participate in the synthesis of heme, essential for the transport of oxygen throughout the body and adequate blood oxygen levels.[4] Wow, low hormones and "iron-poor blood" can result from distressed mitochondria? With their well-being so pivotal to your energy and your overall health, these guys absolutely must have fair working conditions—or else.

How Energy Gets Made

How does all this "magic" happen—how exactly do your mitochondria work? Their energy-making process is called *cellular respiration*. The technical name for the conversion of food and oxygen into energy, cellular respiration occurs over and over in every single mitochondrion like an internal assembly line in which multiple processes happen one after another. It starts with carbon: At the most elemental level—you Star Trek fans will love this—you are a carbon-based life-form. All the food you eat eventually breaks down into a bunch of carbon molecules in sugars, amino acids, and fats, which cross into your cells and then into your mitochondria. Once inside, these molecules enter into a series of reactions known as the Krebs cycle (aka the assembly line). First, they get converted into charged (think electrified) particles, which then get ushered across the inner mitochondrial membrane through a series of chemical reactions. During this process, the molecules become increasingly excited or "charged." The charged particles are like hot potatoes increasing in heat as they jump from one level of charge to the next. In the final step of the Krebs cycle, a positive hydrogen ion gets stripped off enzymes, and when combined with a waiting oxygen molecule, the high energy molecule ATP is produced.

Like most energy production, this process generates byproducts, including carbon dioxide, water, heat, and some nasty pollutants called *reactive oxygen species* (ROS), which are like exhaust from your car's engine. As with your car, mitochondria have their own "catalytic converters" that transform toxic products generated during the combustion process into less harmful compounds. In this case, when rogue electrons (negatively charged molecules) meet oxygen along the production line, ROSs—which include free radicals you have likely heard of—are spewed out. ROSs, including free radicals, are the culprits that drive the oft-mentioned phenomenon of oxidative stress, which is damage done at the cellular level when ROSs outpace our antioxidant capacity, often implicated in aging and chronic disease.

While they can be damaging, ROSs don't fully deserve their "bad guy" reputation. When present in small amounts they play positive roles, acting as signaling molecules that help to maintain cellular health. It's when they are produced *in excess* as a result of your energy factories having to work way too hard, or some part of the "car engine" malfunctioning, that they do their damage. An overproduction of ROS becomes damaging to the mitochondria and may eventually cause them to induce *apoptosis*, a type of cellular death in which the cell or cell components literally explode. A profusion of damaged mitochondria and cells being blown apart is not what you want; this is when cell fragments can enter your circulation and generate more inflammation, and even impair brain function. So how do you prevent ROSs from trashing the place? Luckily, your mitochondria typically have plenty of antioxidants close at hand, allowing them to keep ROSs in balance—enough of them to perform their signaling duties but not too many that they cause harm. But when any part of your mitochondrial supply chain gets messed up—delivering the wrong materials at the wrong time to the assembly line, or too much of the "right" materials, which can overload the assembly line—these "powerhouses of the cell" can become "powerhouses of disease."

Your Mitochondria Are Mighty Flexible

Perhaps our brief overview of the Krebs cycle took you back to your high school biology class for a moment, and you recalled the basic formula that food molecules (from eating) combined with oxygen (from breathing) equals energy. While this formula is fundamentally accurate, it's a little too simplistic. There is a subtle nuance of your energy assembly line that most of us were never taught.

Mitochondria have the ability to process different fuels in slightly different ways to produce ATP. A single mitochondrion can process three different fuel substrates, all of which carry carbon atoms: glucose or other simple sugars from carbohydrates, amino acids from protein, or fatty acids and/or ketone bodies from fats. To use your car engine as an example again, in a car, there is strict delineation: It either runs on gasoline or diesel, and pity the hapless driver who gets them mixed up at the pump! But your mitochondria have a special gift: They are flexible, not fixed in their ability to use different fuels.

Your digestion system is brilliantly designed to process all of these fuel sources in a specific order. Picture a plate of salmon (protein and a bit of fat), some spinach (glucose and fiber), and sweet potatoes (glucose from starch plus fiber) all drizzled with olive oil (fat). All three types of fuel need to eventually make it into the energy-making assembly line, but they don't come in simultaneously. The simple carbohydrates are broken down the fastest. Starch, a more complex carbohydrate, takes a bit longer to break apart, but both become glucose, which is absorbed quickest of all fuels, so your mitochondria typically process this first. Proteins have to be digested and broken down into amino acids before they can be absorbed from your gut, so they arrive for processing in cells later; even then, they have to be transformed into glucose or another compound called *pyruvate* via a process known as glycolysis before they can enter the energy assembly line. Ingested fats usually arrive last, as they are absorbed totally differently through the gut wall; they enter your lymph system and take a circuitous route around your body to eventually get into your bloodstream and then your cells. Since this example of an "ideal" meal contains whole, unprocessed ingredients with the fiber intact—like the spinach and the sweet potato—your digestion and absorption of the different components takes place slowly, so that your mitochondria don't become overwhelmed by too many fuels arriving at once. The "wholeness" of these foods, requiring a lot of breakdown into components, literally acts as stoplights and speed bumps as the food molecules vie to make it up the on-ramps and onto your mitochondrial energy highway; it allows them to merge in gradually.

This ability of mitochondria to switch between several different fuel sources to generate ATP with ease is called *metabolic flexibility*. Metabolic flexibility is the cornerstone of a healthy energy system and indeed of all health and longevity: Without it, your energy production can start to break down. Having metabolic flexibility ensures that your mitochondria can keep your body and brain powered, even when one type of fuel runs out, such as when supplies of glucose are low or, more mundanely, every night when you are asleep and not eating. By design, your mitochondria shift to a slow burn at night, doing repair work and taking it easy like any workers would hope to after a busy day. With no new food to process, they would normally shift to using excess fuel that's been stored in your fat cells. When there's no incoming food (hopefully you aren't sleep eating!), these stored fats are released into your circulation as free fatty acids (FFAs)—think of them as your slow burn fuel. Under certain conditions, your mitochondria can *also* burn ketones, a special type of fat produced in your liver from fatty acids when sugar supplies stay very low for a significant block of time, such as when you have not consumed carbohydrates in your diet, have not eaten for about twelve hours, or have burned up all your stored sugars (glycogen) through intense exercise. Ketones, as you'll learn soon, are highly supportive in your quest for mitochondrial health and mental clarity too, but probably not in the way you think.

You might compare this "flex fuel" system to a hybrid car. While it is running on gasoline (glucose), the battery is getting recharged (fat storage), and this stored electrical energy is available to draw from once the gas is gone or the gas engine is off. Likewise, at night, when you are not eating, mitochondria draw on your "battery" power in the form of FFAs and/or ketones to create ATP.

Having the ability to use a full range of fuel sources offers a host of benefits. First, it means that when you stop eating at the end of the day, you don't keel over—your body simply burns stored fuel. Second, it means that your brain, which is quite a glucose hog normally, can still function in the lean times too. In fact, you make ketones during "tough times" to keep your brain neurons alive, not for anything else. We will return to this subtle but very important point again and again. You make ketones for your brain neurons when glucose is running low. Unlike all other cells in our body (except red blood cells), our brain can't use liberated free fatty acids to make energy (they literally cannot get into the brain easily and in a timely fashion), but it can use both ketones and butyrate, the latter made by your gut buddies, to make ATP.[5]

Third, mitochondrial flexibility allows your energy system to accommodate periodic fluctuations in food source and availability. Think of your ancestors—the hunter-gatherers from whom you evolved. When they had a successful hunt or forage, perhaps after some tough and hungry days, they didn't just have a nibble, they'd eat their fill. They learned to process a big influx of one kind of fuel—say the protein from wild game or a rush of carbohydrates from a wild berry bounty or beehive—and then, once that was finished, switch fuels on a dime and start burning stored fats in the lean times that inevitably followed. This skill set of metabolic flexibility is innate to your mitochondria's design but can be lost when you consume refined and ultra-processed food too frequently—and worse, combine that with a sedentary lifestyle.

Returning your mitochondrial function to good working order is the key to restoring flexibility and making more energy.

From Flexible to Stuck

Now let's contrast our "whole" meal of salmon, sweet potato, and spinach to many of the foods we consume as a part of our modern diet. Our food supply today often delivers "food-like food" in which, stripped of fiber during the manufacturing process, simple sugars, fats, and proteins arrive on our plates *predigested*, a term used by Dr. David Kessler in his book *Fast Carbs, Slow Carbs*. (Fun fact: The term *predigested* was first used by Kellogg's to describe their corn flakes as the world's first predigested meal.) In this state, all of the various fuel sources are prepackaged for hyper absorption simultaneously and hit your bloodstream and liver in a sudden "rush hour." Compounding the problem, our diet is brimming with fructose. Fructose is the sugar in fruit, corn, and beets and while that sounds fine and dandy (hey, those things are all natural, right?) your body did not evolve to consume it in great quantity (it also happens to be omnipresent throughout our food supply in the form of high-fructose corn syrup). Unlike glucose, which is absorbed directly into your bloodstream, fructose is absorbed from your gut in a direct shot into your liver, where it gets converted into the fatty acid palmitate and immediately released into your bloodstream. So, now you've got free fatty acids and glucose arriving simultaneously at your mitochondria, which normally wouldn't happen—remember, fats that you eat always take the "long road" home, circulating in the lymph system after they're absorbed through the gut via fat transport molecules called chylomicrons before they get into your bloodstream. But consuming a lot of fructose, which produces palmitate, means both free fatty acids and glucose hit your mitochondria simultaneously.

Since fats require a different process for ATP conversion than glucose does, the assembly line starts to jam up even before other fuel sources (such as proteins) arrive. The result: mitochondrial gridlock.[6]

Up until one hundred years ago, this gridlock wasn't an issue, as "whole foods" were eaten, well, whole, giving your mitochondria time to process each source of fuel efficiently. Our modern traffic jam has real consequences on energy production—when everyone is jockeying to nudge onto the mitochondrial freeway, fender benders and road rage (those ROS guys) crop up and little to no energy is produced. No wonder your energy crashes after eating fast food, or that power smoothie, or a typical Western high-fat, high-protein, high-carb meal—there are literally multiple crashes happening on your energy-producing freeway! Now, multiply this problem with the fact that most of us are busy digesting and processing food for up to sixteen hours a day, every day—the road never has a chance to clear.

The Paradox of "Mono" Diets

I've studied this conundrum a lot over the years, musing and writing about the conditions our mitochondria need in order to do their best work. And one paradox that has stood out to me, odd as it seems: So often the "balanced diet" recommended by nutritionists causes weight gain and energy loss, while rather more extreme eating protocols seem to offer successful results. Let me explain. If you've followed my writing, you've seen me muse about the benefits and deficits of various diet programs. Over my career, I've seen a wild panoply of restricted diets touted, each of whose proponents swear is the *only* way to get healthy, energized, and lean. Just a smattering of them: the Duke rice diet (yes, basically all you eat is rice); the egg diet (you guessed it); the cabbage soup diet; the

original Atkins diet (high-fat, low-carb); the more recent carnivore diet (which is really a modified Atkins diet, high-protein,
low-carb); the no-oil vegan diets like Eat to Live or Forks Over
Knives (which are high-carb, low-protein, and low-fat); the keto
diet (80 percent fat, ultra-low-carb, and low-protein); and the
Okinawan diet (85 percent sweet potatoes). Here's the thing: *They
all work.* They really do. (Go ahead and mock me on Twitter about
this! I can take it.) All of these diets produce weight loss in overweight and obese individuals, they all reverse diabetes, and in
general restore that get-up-and-go, albeit some faster or slower
than others. Wildly different, but the same results.

So what's happening? I submit to you that their success comes
from making things really easy on the mitochondria. You pick
one substrate and stay with it and your mitochondria can practically do their work on autopilot. It's called mono dieting, and
in addition to limiting the fuel substrate, you eat on a predictable schedule—because, well, you're on a diet, right? No matter
what calorie source you choose, pure carbs, or pure protein, or
pure fat, this form of diet almost always works in the short-term.
Plus, the monotony of solely eating one type of food usually slows
down your consumption of that food too, because you get bored,
and over time, eat less, and so you lose weight. (The phenomenon
of wildly different diets having similar effects was even given a
humorous twist in the book *The Gluten Lie: And Other Myths About
What You Eat,* by Alan Levinovitz, who took other authors' words
of praise for their own wildly different diets and made up a ficti-
tious diet, the UNpacked diet.)

Sadly, these diets almost always fail long-term. It's nearly
impossible to keep up the mono diet constraints; and once you
again start forcing mitochondria to deal with a mixture of fuel
sources—because, boredom eventually hits and you crave nor-
malcy again—sure enough, the weight starts coming back and

energy levels tank. Why? I submit that any mono diet rarely promotes or engenders mitochondrial flexibility. In fact, in my own practice, I have seen followers of all the mono diets I mentioned above develop insulin resistance, prediabetes, and/or full-on diabetes. The phenomenon happens like clockwork (and reliably enough that one has to wonder, is this phenomenon what fuels our search for "diet foods" and hacks?).

Although I don't recommend following any of these diets for the long-term, we can learn a valuable lesson from them: Initially, the easier you make things on your mitochondria, and the less juggling they have to do between carbs, proteins, or fats, the better they restore their function. Stay with me, because in Part II, this principle will become an integral part of your turnaround plan. But first, I want you to know just a little more about the optimal conditions needed for mitochondrial energy production.

Meet Your Supporting Players

Like a state-of-the-art factory, your mitochondria's assembly lines are finely tuned. There's a lot that goes into making a superior-grade product (ATP), and if there are any glaring breaks in the supply chain, production levels plummet. Your mitochondria are mighty strong, but they are also mighty sensitive! Besides needing the raw materials from food to make ATP, several other conditions must be met for the facility to crank out energy so you feel and function your best. Even though this point got left out of biology class (because we didn't know back then! Heck, we didn't know this even a few years ago!), a robust and well-fed microbiome is one of those conditions.

Your gut buddies send postbiotic messages—in the form of butyrate, hydrogen, hydrogen sulfide, and more—that in various ways modulate mitochondrial function for the better. To get very technical about one of these, hydrogen "donates" protons into the hot potato process, amplifying the energy buildup, and simultaneously provides a protective effect to mitochondria. Butyrate, as we'll soon see, signals your mitochondria to stay high functioning. Postbiotic compounds, like hydrogen and hydrogen sulfide, can even deliver fuel in a pinch. In short, it's essential to ensure that communication lines between your gut buddies and their sister mitochondria stay open.

There are three more important links in the supply chain that need to be in place for energy production, but tend to go missing in our modern lifestyle. The first is full-spectrum light. Washington University professor Dr. Gerald Pollack posits that natural light "excites" semi-crystalline water in cells, almost like charging a liquid battery. While for our purposes, you don't need to understand every biochemical pathway of energy production in mitochondria, this is in line with other research describing how near-infrared light (invisible to the eye but occupying 40 percent of the natural light spectrum) and visible red light (the light you see at sunrise and sunset) actually control ATP production by changing water movement within mitochondria using quantum mechanics![7] Other researchers in the field of photo biomodulation (using light wavelengths to induce biological effects) have shown that infrared and red wavelengths of light break up excess nitric oxide that would otherwise bog down ATP production.[8] This is partly why red light therapy has become popular; it's also why walking on the beach at dawn or sunset makes you feel so great. As you'll learn in Chapter 6, sunlight carries important data that tells your mitochondria what time it is and when to do what jobs; it is the major cue to the circadian clock in your body that regulates much of your functioning, including energy production. When light hits your eyes, a protein in your retinas called *melanopsin* communicates with a part of your brain called the *suprachiasmatic nucleus*

(SCN), the master clock that regulates your circadian rhythm. Meanwhile, when sunlight hits your skin, melanin (the complex polymer of tyrosine that gives your skin its color) converts the light energy into ATP, much as chlorophyll does in a plant.[9] The upshot for you: The more you expose your eyes and skin to natural light throughout the day, the better your energy system can work.

After light, the second mitochondrial must-have is a solid infrastructure. Just like a good production facility needs a well-constructed building, your mitochondria need superbly healthy membranes to do their best work. The outer mitochondrial membranes allow the fuel sources to enter in, and the inner ones are the canvas through which electrons flow smoothly from one energy level to the next. These membranes are composed of a variety of lipids, or large-molecule fats, and chief among them are a diverse category of fats called *phospholipids*. Phospholipids give membranes their integrity—a kind of flexible strength that ensures they protect the contents inside the organelle while also easily allowing the exchange of nutrients and information.[10,11]

The most important of all the mitochondrial membrane lipids is *cardiolipin*; it is essential for inner membrane mitochondrial formation and function. To make it, you need to have enough of an essential omega-6 short-chain fatty acid called *linoleic acid*. (The word *essential*, in this context, means that your body can't manufacture it; you have to get it from food.) Unfortunately, the profusion of industrially modified fats called *trans fats* in the typical modern diet has created a big hitch in this production cycle. Such fats, made by hydrogenating seed-based oils so they are solid at room temperature—think Crisco—are technically banned from processed foods but slip into most packaged foods via a loophole and are still present in fast food and most restaurant chain cooking oils. When you eat them (and it's easy to do so, as amounts lower than 0.5 g per serving don't have to be legally listed on food labels,

nor most bulk foods supplying schools, cafeterias, and other insti-
tutions) they not only make the membranes unyielding and stiff,
they kick out cardiolipin, and insert themselves in up to 20 percent
of its lipid real estate![12] With a 20 percent reduction in the membrane space and function taken up by trans fats, it's no wonder a
diet loaded with processed foods and fast foods leaves you so wiped
out. You've taken 20 percent of your energy production capability
off-line, just by eating the wrong kinds of fats. And if that wasn't
enough, our modern diet is loaded with linoleic acid, primarily
from seed oils like corn, canola, and soybean. But that ought to
help you make more cardiolipin, right? Sadly, here too the Goldilocks rule applies: none is bad, some is great, more is horrible. Too
much linoleic acid paralyzes the entire cardiolipin-making process. But don't panic. Since these membranes are constantly being
repaired, you'll kick these bad guys to the side of the road by eating
the right fats in the right proportions.

Okay, we've got light, we've got membrane lipids, now we need
one more key ingredient for proper mitochondrial support: the
master antioxidant, melatonin. Though this hormone is known for
its very important sleep-inducing effects, its purview is far bigger
than that; it is the master mitochondrial-protecting hormone,
perhaps even the center player in the sophisticated protective system of antioxidants that keep ROS in check.[13] While melatonin is
synthesized in the pineal gland in your brain and secreted upon
proper light signals to your master circadian clock regulator, the
SCN, there's also a lot of *subcellular* melatonin inside your mitochondria, which contain melatonin receptors. There, it patches up
the damaging leaks so your mitochondria don't lose efficiency and
it helps to prevent unnecessary mitochondrial death. Consider it
your mitochondria's BFF. It's hypothesized that this subcellular
melatonin is produced in response to the near-infrared photons
in natural sunlight, another reason that exposure to daylight is so

important.[14] If you live in a city or in a northern climate, getting as much outdoor time as you might need can be frustratingly elusive. The good news is that we can acquire melatonin by eating plants. Yes, plants make melatonin!

You might ask, "What the heck is a plant making melatonin for? It doesn't need to go to sleep!" It turns out that melatonin is used by plants to protect the seeds' and leaves' mitochondria under stressful conditions. Bioavailable melatonin gets soaked up by your cells when you have your fill of mushrooms (the darker the better!) or red wine. And by the way, it's the melatonin in wine, rather than its much-touted polyphenol resveratrol, that gives red wine its health benefits. Over the last decade or so we've all been celebrating resveratrol as the fountain of health—but maybe it's actually the melatonin in their diets that's been keeping those French people in enviable shape for so long!

What's more, multiple staples of the Mediterranean diet, like olive oil, olives, purslane (yes, the weed that's probably growing on your sidewalk right now), and pistachios, all contain significant amounts of melatonin. The lesson? Drown your vegetables in 100 percent olive oil, enjoy mushrooms frequently, top your salads with pistachios, and if you love red wine, enjoy it in moderation—you'll be protecting your mitochondria from the damaging oxidative stress that results from their fatiguing overwork.

You have an elegant design perfectly set up to make copious amounts of energy when the right materials and conditions are in place. Unfortunately, for so many people, this is exactly what is not in place. And there is one final dilemma that's hurting our energy production more than any other. It does not discriminate according to dietary preferences or ideologies; it applies almost universally. It is a state of overwhelm happening on the factory floor and consequently, desperate measures are being taken by the essential workers—your mitochondria—to protect themselves from the onslaught. Dear reader, meet the answer to the overfed, under-powered conundrum.

Mitochondrial Gridlock: A Recipe for Exhaustion

As I was writing this chapter, I made a call to one of my newer patients, Peter, who had been seen by my physician's assistant, Mitsu, a few months earlier. In his seventies, he'd done a lot of "livin'" if that's what you want to call it. He's undergone a qua-druple bypass, survived prostate cancer, and had two autoim-mune disease markers for lupus and rheumatoid arthritis, not to mention a very elevated fasting insulin level, hypertension, high cholesterol, elevated hs-CRP . . . I could go on and on. Mitsu put him on the Energy Paradox Program. Four months later, his auto-immune markers were gone, his hs-CRP normalized, his fasting insulin level plummeted, he stopped taking his statin and high blood pressure drugs, and he lost fifteen pounds. Wow, I thought—this is great! But quite frankly, I wasn't shocked. His results were in line with my expectations.

What really got my attention was when Peter told me that he and his wife had moved to their son's farm in Indiana to help out. They were essentially farmhands—rising at dawn, working all day, lug-ging bales of hay, you get the picture. While I was expecting this septuagenarian to complain of the exhausting lifestyle he was forced to endure, the story he related on the phone that day was the exact opposite: He felt amazing. He could outwork his son, doing physically demanding labor for hours without a rest. Yes, he was delighted with his lab results, but all he could talk about was his newfound energy levels. He couldn't see my face, but I was grin-ning from ear to ear. A seventy-three-year-old kid. That's what I want for you!

Like Peter, 80 percent of my patients have little to no energy when they first walk in the door. When we get to the root of the problem, more than any other issue, I find that they universally lack the metabolic muscle—the flexible strength, as it were—to change up their fuel supplies. They are stuck and stiff; they've lost the mitochondrial flexibility that is their birthright. And when you lose it, you just don't manufacture energy effectively, partly because you are insulin resistant, which means not only do you struggle to burn sugars properly, you are also blocked from using free fatty acids as fuel. Let me give you an example of this. A 2020 study from Stanford University shed light on this dilemma by looking at it through the lens of exercise and "fitness." Exercise is good for everyone, right? And exercise helps reverse insulin resistance, right? Not so, according to this study. Participants who were insulin resistant, aka metabolically inflexible, were unable to derive any benefits from exercise programs or to turn on epigenetic changes in genes that promoted health benefits; only the non-insulin-resistant people benefited from exercise.[15] Now here's the kicker: Many of the folks I see in the same predicament are eating a fairly "balanced" diet, per the nutritional dogma of our time. So what's going on?

To answer that question we need to take a deeper dive into the gridlock that may be occurring right now in your mitochondria. Ever wonder why you seem to run out of energy at about 10 a.m. or midday after a fast food breakfast or lunch? I know you've been told by every diet guru and nutritionist on the internet that the culprit is the "inflammation" from the wheat, dairy, or fried fats that were in those meals, right? Wrong. Those inflammatory foods didn't make you sleepy shortly after eating; inflammation doesn't set in that quickly. And similarly, any trans fats in the food didn't *immediately* stiffen all your mitochondrial membranes. Sure, LPSs can hop on the fat you just ate and cause mitochondrial slowdown, but those too, for the most part, have a slight delay before kicking in, because it is the slow buildup of inflammation in the system, over days, weeks, months, or years, that is more impactful than any single meal. As I mentioned earlier, the acute tiredness you experienced after eating your fast food meal, or your "healthy all-American meal" or power smoothie, was due to something different: You created a logjam at your mitochondrial factories. You overdid it. You gave them too much to do. And smart organelles that they are, they protected themselves, and ground to a stop.

Your Mitochondria's Desperate Measures

Let's continue our freeway analogy to demonstrate in real-world conditions how gridlock thwarts your energy production. Suppose you typically eat three meals and two snacks a day. Each of those meals and snacks are broken down into sugars, proteins, and fats, all arriving at your mitochondria for processing into energy. After your breakfast, it would be rush hour for two to three hours in your own inner highway system as food molecules bombard your mitochondria and, correspondingly, traffic (your energy production) slows to a crawl. But then rush hour starts to wane a little, traffic is about to start moving again, then in comes another rush, the 10 a.m. snack! Oops. You just added more cars to the freeway. Now even the on-ramps are getting clogged, and guess what? Traffic slows to a crawl again. And just as that jam begins to clear, it's lunchtime, and traffic grinds to yet another halt. Wow, no wonder you're flagging by 3 p.m.! Of course, your natural inclination is to grab a pick-me-up, maybe something sweet, so you add a few more cars to the pileup, and now it's dinnertime. Sitting on the couch before bed you're still feeling sluggish so, what the heck, you finish the day with a little treat. *It's been rush hour at your mitochondria for the last sixteen hours.* Now you know what living in LA is like! Lots to do, no way to get there quickly.

To get a different perspective on this energy pileup, let me reference the classic clip from *I Love Lucy* where Lucy and her best friend, Ethel, are working in a candy factory. (You can find it on YouTube. Go ahead, watch it now, I'll wait. Hysterical, right?) Lucy and Ethel's job is to individually wrap and then box the chocolates arriving on a conveyor belt. (Just like your mitochondria have to process each incoming carbon molecule from food and turn it into ATP; in this analogy Lucy and her pal are your mitochondria.) Their boss tells them as they start their shift that if any of the candies make it past them unwrapped, they're fired. As the belt starts, it moves slowly; chocolates come to them at a steady pace, and they can keep up. It's easy work; then all of a sudden, the conveyor speeds up. Candies stream in by the bucketload and start to get past them. They're desperate! They try to eat them, or stuff them in their hats, throw them down their blouses; they need to hide them, and they do—just about. The boss comes back and sees the two workers looking like the cats that ate the canaries; situation handled. (Sort of.) The boss looks around, sees that all the candy is taken care of, says, "You're doing great!" and yells to the conveyor operator: *Speed it up!* Lucy and Ethel look aghast.

This legendary TV clip offers a memorable metaphor for what's happening to your mitochondria. Your assembly-line workers, your mitochondria, try desperately to keep up with all the food that you consume, trying to convert it to energy, but they simply can't move that quickly. So, like Lucy and Ethel shoving the excesses of candy into their blouses, your mitochondria shuttle all the extra calories into fat cells. This is their "first buffer" against the onslaught. *We'll stash them wherever we can, and try to circle back to burn them for energy later.* The result? Forced to juggle storage with production simultaneously, and trying to protect your cells from too many ROSs, your energy production decreases while storage (fat deposits) increases. Sounds familiar, right? You feel tired and fat.

Now, if the conveyer belt overwhelm is occasional, it's not such a big deal. After all, your hunter-gatherer ancestors sometimes got a big feast. Your body can handle that from time to time. But, if the pace keeps up without a break, day after day, you can imagine how stressful that might be on the workers. And don't forget, in real life, most of us aren't gorging on a single fuel substrate like a side of bison (mainly protein) or bushes of ripe berries (carbohydrates), as our long-ago ancestors did. We consume all of them all at once and all the time. So it makes matters even worse. Imagine the boss forcing already overworked Lucy and Ethel to wrap three different kinds of chocolates coming down three conveyer belts and merging into one. Whew, they now have to sort, prioritize, and wrap in the same short space of time. Each wrapping job is slightly different, requiring a unique twist, which pushes them to the brink. Do they walk off the job, or do they figure out a workaround before they completely collapse? Your mitochondria, faced with the volume of food substrates coming in, each one requiring slightly different treatment in the Krebs cycle, must make a similar choice. There are only so many places to put all those chocolates to wrap later.

And it's serious. Because just like Lucy and Ethel's blouses reach a bursting point, so do your fat cells. You see, you only have a limited number of fat cells (did you know that?), and they can only hold so much fat or they literally burst. Yes, I did say *burst*. And when fat cells burst, they scatter debris and mitochondria, which, you guessed it, provokes inflammation. So stuffing the fat cells to bursting point is clearly not a good long-term plan, especially since the onslaught does not stop. Faced with such a dilemma, your mitochondria pull the emergency brake.

Fuel Everywhere . . . but Not a Drop to Drink

When a continuous input of food causes energy gridlock and fat cells become dangerously overstuffed, your mitochondria turn to their next defense against being overwhelmed: They create waxy, complex lipids called *ceramides* to help strengthen the fat cell walls as best they can. You may have seen ceramides touted by beauty brands; they're used in skin creams to plump up your complexion and diminish the look of wrinkles. How do they achieve such a miraculous effect? They thicken cell walls of fat cells so that, as the contents increase, the fat stays in without bursting. (Like Lucy reinforcing the seams of her blouse so it doesn't pop open.) They are actually a good defense mechanism for occasional use—the aforementioned feasting on berry bushes in their prime, as your ancestors would have done.

But there's a cruel modern twist to this scenario. There are different kinds of ceramides; some pretty good, some horrible. The horrible ones are made from a fat called *palmitate* or *palmitic acid* (the nomenclature is C:16). The major source of palmitate in your diet, which I mentioned before, is *fructose*, the main form of sugar in fruit, honey, high-fructose corn syrup, and half of the sugars in good old table sugar. Since fructose sneaks into the average Western diet in excessive amounts, your liver has premade lots of palmitate for you, which, in the situation of mitochondrial overwhelm, arrives at your poor overworked mitochondria ready to help.[16]

When ceramides stiffen the walls in your fat cells, a second effect occurs. Their presence slows down the arrival of raw materials feeding into the assembly line. Sounds like a wise idea, right? Conveyer belts are overflowing, a total logjam is imminent, so we better stop the materials from even arriving at the factory floor so the workers can have a fighting chance of catching up! Now, here is where the hormone insulin enters the story.

Insulin, made by the pancreas, acts as a key to unlock the cell membrane to move sugars and proteins out of your bloodstream and into your cells. As I tell my patients, insulin is a salesman who sells sugar and protein to the customer cells; he or she must get that sugar out of the bloodstream or they don't get paid. (Fatty acids, by contrast, don't need it to enter the cell.) So, insulin the salesman rings the doorbell on your cells' doors. But the presence of ceramides blocks the ability of insulin receptors on your cells to detect insulin outside. They can't hear the doorbell ring. This is a problem, because without picking up the signal, they don't "open up" to let sugars and proteins in for processing.

Now, that would seem like a good thing given the overwhelm, right? A little break gives your mitochondria time to catch up on the backlog. That might be fine, occasionally (there's that word again), but what happens if you keep eating and the food keeps entering your bloodstream? You can't stop the food arriving at the factory door. So instead, your pancreas pours *more* insulin (more salesmen) into the bloodstream, trying to signal louder and louder to your cells to open up the doors. Yet, there's so much ceramide insulation that your cells can't hear the doorbell, no matter how hard and how often it's rung. The result is a condition known as *insulin resistance*; and what has been little understood until a recent spate of research is that the thicker your ceramide level in the cell walls (which we can measure by checking ceramide levels in your blood), the more insulin your body produces to try to shove sugar and proteins into cells. With less fuel getting into cells, energy production slows and sputters . . . while blood sugar and insulin levels continue to climb. In fact, although there are different forms of ceramides, it's the C:16 formed from fructose becoming palmitate that's the real culprit starving your cells.[17,18,19,20]

But the problem gets worse. If you've been paying attention, you might ask, surely free fatty acids could come into the cell (they don't need insulin to get into cells) to restart energy production, could they not? After all, you have tons of them waiting in the fat storage spaces. But, here's the cruel gut punch (excuse the pun): The presence of insulin in the bloodstream tells your fat cells *not* to liberate fats. This too has evolutionary precedent: When you got your feast of bison or berries, a surge of insulin would direct those sugars and proteins into the fat cells to store for a rainy day by releasing the fat-storing enzyme lipoprotein lipase and blocking the fat-releasing enzyme hormone-sensitive lipase, so fat liberating would be on pause. Think about it—if insulin is high, it's time to store fat, not use it. You wouldn't do both. Insulin, in other words, blocks you from burning stored fat while simultaneously making it easier to store fat.

In a normally functioning system with metabolic flexibility, when sugar and proteins are not going into your bloodstream, because you had stopped eating, your insulin level would fall, the fat-releasing enzyme hormone-sensitive lipase would be released (technically, it would be unblocked by insulin levels falling), free fatty acids would flow out of your fat cells to your other cells in need of fuel, you'd make a few ketones in your liver from those same fats just for your brain; and then twelve hours or so later, breakfast arrives and the system goes back to the start again. That's metabolic flexibility. When you are chronically tired, which, may I remind you, is most likely why you are reading this book, I can assure you this metabolic flexibility is not happening in your cells. Now you're in a dilemma: You've got plenty of stored fat to use as fuel, but no way to get to it, because that high insulin level won't let you. Water, water everywhere and not a drop to drink! Which means you feel tired, sluggish, hungry, and hangry, and you start to become increasingly more insulin resistant, which soon leads to a diagnosis of prediabetes, which then leads to diabetes. (By the way, calling you a prediabetic is like calling you female readers "a little bit pregnant.")

Incidentally, this mechanism explains why ultra-low-carb and/ or high-fat diets generally make you feel awful when you start them. Call it the keto flu or the Atkins blues—your energy levels tank, your brain stops functioning, and you feel like, well, crap. Chronically high insulin levels don't change overnight, and your fat cells are prevented by high insulin from liberating free fatty acids for you to burn and also turn into ketones—even though all the books say that's what should happen. They didn't account for insulin blocking that action. It can take weeks for insulin levels to come down so you can feel normal let alone more energized, during which so many people become utterly demoralized, and give up.

I have a secret for you: Even *with* this issue of insulin resistance, you can make the transition to burning fat as fuel relatively painlessly. Remember how I said your gut buddies can help make fuel, in a pinch, for your mitochondria? Turns out that if you had only given your microbiome what it needed, they would have made butyrate, hydrogen, hydrogen sulfide, and methane that your mitochondria and your brain could have used as an alternative fuel during this transition. But you didn't, did you? Additionally, a few small tweaks to your diet can help protect you against the harmful effects of ceramides. Olive oil and DHA and EPA (long-chain fatty acids from fish oil) protect against your body making ceramides and help restore mitochondrial function,[21,22] while the ketone BHB produced from butyrate can lower ceramides.[23] Soon I'll show you how to include all of your gut buddies' favorite foods in your diet.

Uncoupling: A Last Resort

Okay, before we move on, let's revisit Lucy and Ethel one last time. Despite the fact that they've been stuffing all the extra chocolates anywhere they can find, as fast as they can, let's suppose they still can't keep up with the assembly line. What then? Well, by this time

Lucy and Ethel are exhausted, they're sweating and irritable, so they say, forget it, we have to protect ourselves, we're working too hard. They start to let the chocolates go by without the wrapper.

Now believe it or not, your overworked mitochondria do the same thing. It's called *mitochondrial uncoupling* or *decoupling*, or *mitochondrial proton leak*, and in simple terms, it describes the mitochondria making an active choice *not* to make ATP out of every last carbon molecule that arrives for processing. Instead, they let some "leak by" without generating any ATP. Making energy is hard work, and as you'll recall, it's a process that generates by-products—including heat and those ROSs that can damage mitochondria. Your mitochondria make the call to actively dump some of these "hot potatoes" to keep from getting "burned," literally. And just so we're clear, mitochondria do this all the time, even in the best of times; but when overwhelmed like poor Lucy, they do it a lot. That means that the more calories you eat, the more often you eat them, and the more varieties of macronutrients you eat, the less energy you make.

Want more bad news? All this work you throw at your mitochondria wears them out. Not only do these tired workers create less ATP, they actually start to *use more ATP than they make*.[24] This mitochondrial dysfunction is at the root of all degenerative diseases, like dementia, heart failure, and exhaustion; no wonder the neurons (dementia) or heart muscle cells (heart failure) are dying. They're not just holding on for dear life, their energy has been sucked out by damaged mitochondria.

Furthermore, as mitochondria get damaged, our cellular immune system starts to recognize them for who they are, that is, *bacteria*, and sets out to destroy them. And that destruction produces inflammation. I hope that got your attention! "Holy cow, if one of my cells dies because my mitochondria are messed up, my immune system will think I'm being invaded by bacteria?" The answer is yes! That's why all of this, in the end, is so important. The theories that "all disease is inflammation" and "all disease is mitochondrial dysfunction" become one unified theory.

So, is there a solution for you? There are actually two. One solution is to simply eat less so your energy system isn't overwhelmed all the time. Yup, that's the typical "go on a diet" solution to the problem. Your mitochondria are temporarily happy, but your energy is still not being produced—and boy will you feel grouchy. As you have probably experienced, it's a short-term fix that doesn't last.

So, solution number two. In order to get production up to demand, Lucy and Ethel get help; three conveyor belts are added, and eight more factory workers are brought to the assembly-line floor. Your mitochondria "hire" more workers through a process called mitogenesis. But there are usually only two ways to induce mitochondrial replication: through fasting and/or exercise. On the Energy Paradox Program, I'm going to teach you a third way to add more energy workers to the line. That action plan is in Part II, and it involves changing the working conditions in the factory. Give the workers shorter shifts and lots of break time, improve morale with help from the microbiome, and you'll attract more workers to the assembly line, sharing the work evenly. Believe it or not, you actually have the resources ready and waiting in your fat stores, and with a few tweaks to your gut, you will be getting that energy surge in no time at all.

But before we do that, we have one more very important stop to make: your foggy, fuzzy, worn-out brain.

ENERGY MYTH #4: **Help! My Thyroid Has Given Out on Me**

Very frequently, patients arrive to see me saying they feel dulled, dragging, and somewhat depressed, and (smart patients that they are) they feel their thyroid function might have something to do with it. But their doctor ran tests and said their levels seem normal—so what gives? The truth is, there is an epidemic of hypothyroidism (low thyroid) occurring, and it can have a major effect on your energy levels, your mental focus, your mood, and even your cholesterol levels. But what's little known is that the function of your thyroid hormones also has something to do with conditions in your gut.

Your thyroid gland produces the thyroid hormones T4 and T3 (levothyroxine and liothyronine, respectively) that regulate your body's basal metabolic rate (BMR), literally the number of calories you burn to maintain your life and generate heat. By now, many practitioners know to check thyroid function with bloodwork (it's a good idea to do this annually even if you are well), but what thyroid tests can't assess is whether or not your body is getting thyroid hormone where it's needed. That means that your thyroid levels could fall within the "normal" range, but there is still dysfunction going on.

A quick review: Your thyroid gland makes thyroid hormones by extracting iodine from the blood and incorporating it into T4 and T3. The hypothalamus secretes thyroid-stimulating hormone (TSH) to tell the thyroid gland to produce thyroid hormones. I use TSH as the measurement of how much the receptors for the thyroid hormone in the brain are picking up the presence of active forms of the thyroid hormone, free T4 and free T3. Now, if your microbiome is out of whack, so may be your thyroid function, because you need a healthy microbiome to convert the thyroid hormone precursors into their usable forms. Moreover, gut inflammation can raise cortisol, which, in turn, can suppress thyroid hormones. (It goes both ways: Those thyroid hormones then help the gut's tight junctions work properly.) If your gut becomes leaky, as I have published, it can cause the autoimmune form of hypothyroidism, Hashimoto's thyroiditis.

Low thyroid has become endemic today because of poor gut health, the thyroid-harming effects of endocrine disruptors, and by the way that pesticides in particular block the receptors for thyroid hormones on all cell membranes of the body. You're being hit with a double blow: Your body is hampered to make the right amounts of thyroid hormone and simultaneously blocked from getting it where it's needed!

To add insult to injury, our "healthy" diet has contributed to a deficit of iodine, which is required to make thyroid hormones. In the past, we got sufficient iodine from ocean fish and shellfish, but today (unless you live in coastal Maine, maybe), by and large we don't. Back in the early 1900s, there was such an epidemic of hypothyroidism as Americans moved inland from the coasts that the federal government mandated iodine be put into table salt— yes, the little girl with the umbrella on the blue package—and it by and large resolved the problem. Alas, our sophisticated foodie tastes have led us to other salts, like pink salt (Himalayan salt) and sea salt, which are both iodine-free. There is an easy solution to this dilemma; use iodized sea salt or add iodine-containing spirulina or chlorella or seaweed to your diet.

I treat many patients with all forms of hypothyroidism. And one of the things I do for all of them is look closely at TSH. Since TSH drives the production of thyroid hormones, when it's low, it means the brain sensor is saying, okay, I've got plenty of thyroid, I don't need to send a signal to make more! (Low levels are 0 or 1 or max 2 uIU/ml—not the 3.5 or 4 or even 4.5 that many endocrinologists have told my patients is perfectly fine.) So, I encourage you to ask your doctor to measure TSH, free T4 and free T3, and reverse T3 levels, and pay particular attention to TSH. The first number before the decimal point should be a 1 or a 2. If your TSH is higher than 2.4 uIU/ml, that's your brain saying that it's not getting enough thyroid hormone and it's pushing for more! Please don't rely on simply checking T4 and T3; these are not the active forms.

For low thyroid patients (whether autoimmune-induced or not), my approach to restore thyroid function is to repair the leaky gut while restoring a diverse microbiome; add iodine back into the diet, restore vitamin D levels, and only then, if needed, I may write a prescription for thyroid hormones to get levels restored while we are continuing to improve the foundation of thyroid health. These simple interventions—and sometimes it really is as basic as switching to iodized sea salt—typically resolve thyroid malfunction.

CHAPTER 5

———

INFLAMED AND ENERGY STARVED

THE TIRED MODERN BRAIN

When new patients arrive at my office with complaints of feeling exhausted, they often share that previous practitioners have suggested their symptoms are "all in their head." Their doctors had found nothing out of the ordinary in these folks' bloodwork and simply came to the conclusion that nothing was physically wrong with them.

So it puzzles these patients when, after running my own battery of tests, I too conclude: "It's in your head." But I don't mean to dismiss their symptoms. Just the opposite: I'm acknowledging a very real physiological phenomenon that is impacting the function of their brain, and it is responsible for the fogginess, shortened attention span, and moodiness these patients experience. All of these symptoms—and more—make up a state of mild cognitive impairment I've come to call the *inflamed, starving brain.*

When you feel you "just don't have it in you," it's often because, like the rest of your body, your brain is suffering from inflammation. In addition, your brain is also very likely "overfed and underpowered," struggling hard to meet its energy needs. The neurological fatigue and fogginess that ensues from this combination carries over into your whole being, and it becomes hard to know whether your tired body is dragging your mindset down with it or vice versa.

In my years of tending to patients who are of retirement age and beyond, I've gotten well accustomed to reports of foggy brain and slower, more muddled thinking. But something has shifted in the last few years—the profile of these patients now skews younger. Women and men in their forties, thirties, and sometimes younger who complain of fatigue also talk about brain fog. When I ask how they're handling their work or multiple demands of family and life, they look concerned or downright upset. "It feels like I'm lagging mentally, I can't keep up with my work," they might say. Or, "I can't concentrate like I used to." Or, "Do I have adult-onset ADHD? Should I take Ritalin?" They might experience higher levels of stress or anxiety than before, endure bouts of low mood, or have trouble falling or staying asleep (which makes all of the other problems feel much worse!). If you're experiencing low energy, chances are you've gotten up close and personal with some of these cognitive symptoms as well.

Sleep Your Way to Brain Health

Along with unmanaged stress, mediocre sleep is another piece of the inflamed, starving brain puzzle. As I outlined in *The Longevity Paradox*, deep sleep is of vital importance because it's your brain's "wash cycle" opportunity, when it clears out all the inflammatory compounds that build up over the course of the day. The lymph-containing *glymphatic system* in your brain literally sweeps away brain-inflaming junk and debris when you're in deep sleep, which usually occurs early in the sleep cycle. This is one reason why you shouldn't eat too close to bedtime—digestion diverts blood flow down to the gut instead of giving your brain the resources it needs for its freshening up period. In Part II, I will help you do just that, as you will refrain from eating anything for three hours before bedtime at least once a week (even better, every day).

Moreover, the composition of your microbiome has profound effects on the amount of REM, or rapid eye movement (sometimes called dream sleep), and deep sleep you are likely to get each night. You might have guessed by now, but a diverse, dynamic gut biome actually *helps* you have the deep sleep in which your nightly "brain wash" can take place.[1] Who knew that caring for and feeding your gut bugs help you get a good night's sleep?

The reality is that our energy crisis affects our whole body, including the brain. It's an equal opportunity dilemma. Just like how we can't easily diagnose bodily fatigue with standard blood tests, most health professionals don't have the training and tests to pick up a lack of mental get-up-and-go. Mild but hard-to-shake brain fog typically gets dismissed by the medical establishment—and very unfairly (I've also noticed that women feel more unheard on this issue than men). Though rushed appointments and gender bias may account for some of this dismissal, so do limited diagnostics; subtle neurological inflammation doesn't show up on standard bloodwork. But there are newer tests that *can* detect markers of brain inflammation, and I've seen these markers appear frequently in the bloodwork of people who are functioning, but lagging and dragging through their days. Most, if not all, of these folks also show evidence of leaky gut. In other words, when you have leaky gut and resulting inflammation, then odds are you will have some degree of leaky brain, a condition in which the brain's protective barrier, called the *blood-brain barrier*, is breached by inflammatory agents, resulting in neurological inflammation (or *neuroinflammation* for short).

In this chapter, we'll look at how inflammation in your brain and the resultant kinks in its mitochondrial supply chain can greatly affect your cognitive function. Your brain tops the list of energy-hungry organs: It demands a ton of ATP to function well. All that thinking, processing, and biochemical coordination requires up to 20 percent of your body's total ATP production.[2] In fact, a single human cortical neuron (the "thinking" cell) uses 4.7 billion (yes, billion) molecules of ATP per *second*! By actual weight, your whole brain uses 6 kg (about 13 pounds) of ATP per day, about five times as much as the brain weighs. Because of this need, your brain cells are very densely packed with mitochondria. So, any slowdown at the mitochondrial level is going to have quite an impact neurologically.

And while mild brain fog is easy to rationalize as just a "senior moment," I strongly suggest not overlooking the consequences. We now know that the same factors driving subtle fogginess today can drive more serious cognitive impairment later in life. Neurodegenerative conditions like dementia, Alzheimer's, and Parkinson's disease are extreme expressions of neuroinflammation and mitochondrial dysfunction. These diseases now affect 10 percent of our population—a figure that is expected to double by 2030; furthermore, these devastating diseases are increasingly striking at a younger age. We now suspect that chronic brain fog early in life could mean a higher likelihood of dementia later, which means turning chronic brain fog around when it is still mild has a very high return on your investment. (Literally. In 2018, dementia care cost $277 billion in the US; you or your loved ones will spend $300,000 over a five-year period if you develop it.)

I want you to consider the symptoms of an inflamed and energy-starved brain as an early warning sign. Your brain fog is giving you a valuable heads-up that there may be a break in the energy supply chain, and that some communication glitches need to be rectified, all starting at the level of the gut, the microbiome, and the mitochondria. The good news is, it's never too late to make a difference. It is possible to clear brain fog by feeding your brain what it needs (which, by the way, involves feeding your gut bugs what *they* need) and enjoy the benefits of clear thinking, mental agility, and an improved mood at any age. But first, let's take a closer look at how the brain and gut are connected and what that connection means for your mental wellness.

Your Second Brain

You've likely heard it said that your gut is your second brain. It's a good maxim, but I like to flip it, because who's to say your downstairs "brain" isn't your first brain, and the gray matter inside your head is getting directions from below? As you're discovering in this book, the gut and its microbiome may have *more* to do with how you think, act, and feel than your brain tissue. If that concept seems hard to believe, remember your gut and your brain are engaged in constant communication, with each influencing and helping the other to maintain homeostasis. We've known for some time that this two-way communication runs on a complex network called the gut-brain axis, but only very recently have we zeroed in on how it works, and the clue is in the name upgrade: We now talk about the *microbiota*-gut-brain axis. (Really, these guys do it all!)

This bidirectional axis of information and communication helps to maintain the stability of the gastrointestinal tract and affects your emotions and cognitive function.

You learned previously that your gut is home to 70 to 80 percent of your immune cells, but it is *also* home to more than one hundred million neurons—more than are in your entire spinal cord. These neurons help control digestion, but more important, at least for the purpose of this chapter, they receive and interpret messages from the environment and your microbiome and then communicate that information to the neurons in your "big brain" upstairs. These intestinal neurons add up to what is called your *enteric nervous system.* Research now shows that emotional stress and depression can cause disorders of the digestive system and vice versa. For example, it was long thought that anxiety or depression caused symptoms of irritable bowel syndrome (a chronic condition of diarrhea and/or constipation). But research now shows that cause and effect can be flipped: Stress can change the environment in the intestines while imbalances and irritation in the "roots and soil" also send signals up to the brain that then trigger changes in mood and outlook.[3] This insight helps to explain why the frequency of GI symptoms is increased in children with autism (in fact, cutting-edge research suggests that GI changes and alterations in the microbiome of autistic kids are most likely driving the brain malfunction[4,5]) and sheds light on why patients with schizophrenia often have increased intestinal permeability and declines in intestinal function.[6]

A vast amount of this axis activity is driven by the microbes in the gut. How could it not be, given how much their vast and rich genome drives your overall function and how many messages to your cells they generate, in the form of postbiotic compounds, every single second? While we have known that neurons in the gut "talk" to the brain and produce neurotransmitters like the mood-boosting serotonin, it was a true "holy cow" moment to discover that the neurons play second fiddle to the gut buddies, who are the ones signaling to those neurons, helping them know what to do. Thus, the five pounds of bugs in your "virtual organ," your holobiome, *dramatically* influence the ways that the 4.5-pound organ in your skull carries out its functions.

Research shows that reintroducing helpful gut buddies to the microbiome in the form of a multispecies probiotic can reduce sadness and rumination,[7] and we know that it's the changes to the gut biome in particular that are at play when you are depressed or suffering from brain fog: Your microbiome composition is measurably different.[8] Moreover, certain bacterial strains seem to modulate how your brain works or, as the case may be, doesn't work. A leaky gut and abnormal microbiome are now known to be key drivers of cognitive decline, including dementia. (Important research pioneered by my friend and colleague Dr. Dale Bredesen, the author of *The End of Alzheimer's*, has revealed that the infamous amyloid plaques behind serious cognitive impairment are in fact *made* by the gut biome and can make their way to the brain, where they stimulate more amyloid production.)[9] As I write this, a newly published review of multiple studies declares that prebiotics and probiotics have been found to measurably reduce symptoms of anxiety and depression.[10]

The precise mechanisms behind the communication between your gut buddies and your brain are still being discovered. But we know that the "chatter" of postbiotic signaling compounds—such as the short-chain fatty acids like butyrate and the gasotransmitters you met earlier—can reach the brain via your circulation. Information can also get transmitted directly via your vagus nerve, which acts like a two-way physical "landline" of communication between your gut and your brain. Furthermore, the gut buddies, in addition to making psychoactive compounds themselves, can signal cells in your gut wall to release hormones and peptides that affect your thinking and mood. And as you've already learned, they also determine how "switched on" your inflammatory immune cells are, which then affects your brain. Net result: Your microbes have a lot of control over whether you see the glass half empty or full, how clearly you think (or don't), and even how easy sleep comes at night.

These discoveries are so cutting-edge that your doctor or your therapist may not even be aware of this seismic shift in our understanding of neurological conditions. I've observed firsthand how my friend and colleague Dr. Daniel Amen, one of the world's leading psychiatrists, has shaken up the field of mental health with the revelations that many psychological conditions can be traced to neuroinflammation caused by a disturbance in the gut. It truly is forcing a reevaluation of what we thought we knew to be true about how the brain functions. The good news in all of this? Many of the psychological and neurological issues that affect millions of people today may be able to be prevented, modified, or hopefully reversed by healing the gut and microbiome and, in turn, the brain.

I can't overstate how important these findings are, given the prevalence of depression, anxiety, and cognitive impairment worldwide, the burden of suffering involved, and how many people go untreated and remain unaware of the physical factors contributing to their illness. Indeed, soon, *the first step* when treating depression as well as cognitive issues may well begin with healing the gut wall and restoring the gut ecosystem to its original condition— dynamic and diverse—thus reducing the prevalence of neuro-inflammation.[11]

When I first saw Sarah, a woman in her early forties who suffered from anxiety and depression, she had been taking multiple antidepressant medications for at least ten years. Sarah "knew" that her brain wasn't working well, her attention span was short, and getting through a normal day's work as a teacher took everything she had; yet she loved her job. After a full workup, we discovered that, as I'd suspected, Sarah had multiple markers of inflammation, classic signs of leaky gut and lectin sensitivity. She also carried mutations of the MTHFR genes, which normally code for creating enzymes that attach methyl groups (for you science nerds, that's CH3) to many of the B vitamins that make them active; 50 percent of people carry one or more of these mutations. Sarah had been advised that because she had these mutations, her mood disturbances were simply genetic destiny. Moreover, despite being told that she did not have diabetes or prediabetes, her fasting insulin level was dangerously high, indicating insulin resistance and hence metabolic inflexibility. We put her on the Energy Paradox Program, reduced the lectins in her diet, added in a lot of prebiotic foods to feed her gut buddies, and slowly began shortening the number of hours she ate during the day. Finally, we supplemented her very low vitamin D levels, added a generous dose of the omega-3 DHA, and gave her methylated B vitamins to make up for what was missing with her MTHFR mutations.

Three months into the program, a new Sarah arrived back in the office. With a sheepish smile, she confessed that after a few weeks she had been feeling so "normal" that she and her therapist had started to decrease her two antidepressants and she was now fully weaned from one and down to half the dosage of the other. Her bloodwork showed no markers of inflammation, a normal (nice and high) vitamin D and omega-3 index, and a normal fasting insulin level. Oh, and she lost fifteen pounds! There was such energy in her face and even composure. And here's the kicker: She looked me in the eyes and said, "I forgot what feeling normal felt like. I was walking in a fog and now the fog's lifted!" Working closely with her therapist, we slowly but surely got her off her remaining antidepressant, and today she is medication-free. When you tame inflammation in the body and the subsequent inflammation in the brain the results can truly be profound.

How the Brain Becomes Inflamed

Have you ever taken a few long, deep breaths in a moment of stress and noticed how much better you feel? Anytime you consciously use your breath to calm yourself down, you're accessing your vagus nerve—a nerve that starts at your brain stem and winds its way through your body, coiling itself around your heart and your gut. The vagus nerve plays a critical role in the microbiota-gut-brain axis—it is a key communication channel used for the cross talk between the brain the microbiome.

The vagus nerve is involved in an incredible amount of regulatory activity—it helps to modulate inflammation, regulate your hunger and satiety levels, and monitor your energy needs. Think of it as a landline for microbe-gut-brain chatter; it physically connects one part to the other in communication. The vagus nerve doesn't only send signals downward from the brain; it's a bidirectional nerve pathway that also picks up signals from your gut and broadcasts them upstairs,[12] likely via newly discovered cells called neuropods that project off your gut lining. If these cells detect a leaky gut, the signal is sent to your brain—"It's chaos down here!"— and the brain responds by signaling for your immune system to investigate. And just like that, inflammation is ignited in the gut while simultaneously started in the brain.

While the vagus nerve is the landline of the microbiota-gut-brain axis—an actual cord connecting the two—there is a second, "wireless" kind of network that facilitates communication as well: free-floating inflammatory cytokines that have launched into your bloodstream as a result of leaky gut. These cytokines can cause real trouble when they make their way past another important barrier in your body—the one that protects your brain, also known as the blood-brain barrier. This critical border is made of cells that allow in needed materials—such as glucose, oxygen, amino acids, and hormones, as well as protective gasotransmitters—while keeping unwanted or hazardous matter out. In between the cells of this border are—you guessed it—tight junctions that ensure nothing sneaks through, just like in your intestine. The barrier also has controllable pores called *aquaporins* that move water in and out.

The walls in your intestine and your brain are similar enough that they are susceptible to the same type of breaching from dietary and environmental assaults—and suffer from the same resulting inflammation.[13] For example, its known that the Western diet, high in sugar and saturated fat and low in microbe-feeding fiber, impairs the integrity of the blood-brain barrier and weakens cognition and memory by causing dysfunction in the part of the brain assigned memory duties, the hippocampus.[14] Alarmingly, glyphosate, the leaky-gut-inducing ingredient in Roundup and similar herbicides (see page 152 for more details on this toxin), also has been shown to weaken the blood-brain barrier.[15],[16] Now for the lectins: It has been proved that the loss of brain-barrier integrity may also be caused by P-glycoprotein dysfunction.[17] What are *P-glycoproteins*, you ask? A class of lectins called *aquaporins*. Yes, that's right, the same type of compounds that populate your blood-brain barrier and your gut wall! In nature, aquaporins are found in a variety of plants, including spinach, corn, potatoes, soybeans, green bell peppers, and tobacco. In certain people, a leaky gut and a tendency toward sensitivity to these lectins can cause the immune system to develop antibodies to the *lectin* aquaporins in food . . . which can then lead it to mistakenly attack the aquaporins in the gut wall and brain—via the molecular mimicry we talked about in Chapter 2. Now before you panic about eating spinach, take note: Most of us don't react to the aquaporins in spinach. But in some tricky cases, the sophisticated testing I use in my clinic has revealed that these aquaporin-containing foods are a hidden cause of a patient's leaky gut and brain, and removing them makes a surprisingly big difference.

It is important to recognize that disruptions in the blood-brain barrier and resulting brain inflammation are also related to the epidemic of neurological issues affecting all ages today, from dementia and Alzheimer's to autism, depression, and schizophrenia, as well as some neurological diseases that have an immunologic component like multiple sclerosis. Thus, removing inflammatory chemicals and cleaning up your diet can heal and seal your blood-brain barrier, so it certainly seems worth the effort. Because whether the signals to your brain to "launch the inflammatory defenses!" have come via the landline (your vagus nerve) or wirelessly (cytokines slipping through the blood-brain barrier), the resulting response in our brain can be devastating in both the short- and long-term.

Starved to Death: Neurons Cut Off from Supplies

Your brain contains a number of specialized cells and, quite frankly, a lot of fat. (Yes, you have my permission to call someone you're mad at "a fathead!") Like your gut, the brain has numerous neurons (actually eighty-six billion of them!), which are the cells that are involved in "thinking." The cell bodies of neurons have long branches called *axons*, which develop shorter, more numerous branches called *dendrites*, which extend outward in all directions to come into contact with dendrites projected from the axons of other neurons. Chemical signals jump between them, connecting the neurons, and when neuronal firing happens repeatedly, simply stated, thoughts and memories are formed. Think of your dendrites as circular "satellite" airport terminals connected by trams and walkways (the axons) that extend outward from the main terminal (the neuron), linking one to the next.

Your brain also has its own specialized immune cells called *microglia* as well as supporting cells called *astrocytes*. Think of them as your neurons' bodyguards. Their job is to protect the neurons from harm, and they take this job extremely seriously—like the guards outside London's Buckingham Palace, they stand ready, sworn to protect and defend the queen at all costs. Your microglia and astrocytes help your brain all through your life, nourishing and supporting the neurons and helping to clear the brain of waste and dead cells. They "prune" away dendrites that are weak in order to give healthy ones a better chance, kind of like a gardener tending her roses. They also take care of threats from within (like proteins taking on the wrong form, potentially causing disease, like beta-amyloid or tau proteins) and threats from outside—LPSs, microbes, lectins, and other invasive agents. When your microglia get the news, either via information traveling up the vagus nerve or cytokines entering via the bloodstream, that bad guys are mobilizing and may put the brain at risk, microglia, as an unintended consequence, ramp up their pruning quite aggressively. Sensing that aggressors are coming, the microglia decide to preserve the neurons they surround, no matter the cost. They literally eat away on the dendritic processes extending from the neurons, almost as if the neuron is calling back their outpost troops, telling them to draw safely back inward to the castle. That's bad enough—your dendrites are no longer at full extension, unable to link to other neurons to communicate. But then, the microglia go a step further: They prune back the axon sheaths and surround the pruned neuron, in a sense pulling up the drawbridge to protect the castle, cutting it off from supplies. While it's a defensive move that is essential during an acute emergency like an infection, it's disastrous when it happens all day, every day, as a result of low-grade inflammation starting in your gut.

Let me give you an example of how this kind of inflammation plays out in real life. My patient Ingrid is in her late thirties, a millennial at a high-tech company. She was in a car accident about two years ago. Shortly afterward, she began having a tremor in her left hand. Thinking it was somehow related to the car accident, doctors did brain MRIs, neck MRIs, and shoulder MRIs, all of which came back normal. She saw physical therapists, acupuncturists, and naturopaths, took thousands of dollars of supplements a month (literally), all to no effect. Finally, she was diagnosed with early Parkinson's disease (yes, in her thirties!). She sought out my clinic and we ran our complete battery of tests. As suspected, she not only had leaky gut, but her blood-brain barrier was leaky as well, and she had an immune attack against the neurons in her cerebellum, the movement center of the brain. Even worse, she had the markers for the autoimmune disease often associated with lupus. Her fasting insulin level was high despite having normal fasting blood sugars, which meant that she was metabolically inflexible. Ingrid was suffering from a perfect storm: Not only was she suffering a direct autoimmune attack against her neurons because of her leaky gut and leaky brain, her under-attack neurons were unable to protect themselves and repair due to insulin resistance in her brain (sometimes called *type 3 diabetes*, or diabetes of the brain).

We started her on the Energy Paradox Program, removed lectins from her lectin-rich diet, shortened her eating window, and arranged the next visit and lab recheck in three months. I saw her for that checkup as I was writing this chapter. Her markers for leaky gut were dramatically lowered (though not gone), but her markers for brain inflammation now came back normal. Her fasting insulin was normal. And the best news is that her tremor was much improved. No, it's not gone, but at the time of this writing it has been only three months, and both she and I have a lot of hope and confidence that we can stop it in its tracks.

Ingrid is just an extreme example of what neuroinflammation can do, but even mild brain inflammation can have a significant impact on your well-being. For many people, thinking gets foggy, memory grows faulty, and overall mental processing power takes a nosedive. What's more, starving neurons send you signals that they need food—and fast. And what food do the starving inflamed neurons want? You guessed it: a quick absorbing, fuel-injecting hit of sugar! Remember your brain is dependent on glucose for fuel—yes, it can use ketones and butyrate as I'll soon describe, but in most people today, the brain is "trained" and addicted to respond to glucose. That's what it knows provides instant energy and ATP production. But, if you've been paying close attention, you know that's the last thing your weakened brain needs. So the next time you get a craving for something sweet, consider the death play going on in your brain before reaching for a cookie!

Microglial pruning is also to blame for the sluggish, mentally impaired feeling you get when you're sleep deprived.[18] That's right, a late-nighter can prune your neurons! And the foods you tend to eat when you're sleep deprived—such as simple carbs and sugar—only make matters worse. Back when I used to do all-night infant heart transplant surgeries, I would crave sugars to keep me going. When you endure night after night of poor sleep, you're setting up conditions for more and more unwanted pruning. No wonder I became seventy pounds overweight and had insulin resistance!

We are just beginning to realize how sensitive this protective system in the brain actually is. It responds in real time to subtle inputs, even those from our emotional state. Take stress, for example. It turns out that stressful events switch on overenthusiastic microglial activation, causing them to prune more dendrites than they should.[19] Now the good news is that, usually, when stress abates and anti-inflammatory signals are received from your immune system and from your gut buddies, microglia can dial down their defense and return to repairing and protecting the brain, just as they are now doing in Ingrid's case. But for that to happen, your brain needs to have access to calming, anti-inflammatory compounds, namely short-chain fatty acids and anti-inflammatory gasotransmitters like hydrogen and hydrogen sulfide, which not only turn off the warning signals but also provide our neurons' mitochondria with alternative fuel sources. Thankfully, these gut buddy by-products are able to cross the blood-brain barrier and both nourish the neurons and tame inflammation.[20,21]

Of course, the problem is that today, not only is stress often ongoing and chronic, but the crisis in our roots and soil means that our microbes don't have what they need to make the anti-inflammatory compounds *we* need. For most people, leaky gut, immune system activation, and microbial imbalances mean that more and more inflammatory signals are being sent northward, at the expense of our neurological health.

A robust and diverse gut microbiome will produce adequate butyrate, which is a potent neuroprotector that has been shown to improve age-related memory decline as well as counter anxiety and depression.[22] Butyrate also stimulates the formation of new brain cells[23] and can help the microglia mature and function properly. Indeed, one study showed that germ-free mice, bred to have no microbiome, had scanty and malformed microglia that couldn't work properly, but adding short-chain fatty acids to the mice's drinking water for four weeks normalized these microglial cells, helping them to perform as they should. Similarly, your human brain's bodyguards *need* butyrate and its other fatty acid brethren to stay in peak condition.[24] (And by the way, if you're a parent, you might like to know that butyrate has another saving grace: It helps modulate kids' behavior.[25] A good reason to get them enjoying a full array of fiber at a young age.)

Meanwhile, the postbiotic gases your biome should ideally be making are also critically important for maintaining your brain. As you learned in Chapter 3, lack of adequate hydrogen-producing bacteria has been observed in patients with Parkinson's disease[26]; this is notable because when your neurons are under siege, hydrogen rushes across the blood-brain barrier and protects the mitochondria inside, allowing them to fight back and stay alive. Hydrogen sulfide has an equally impressive array of brain-preserving properties (incidentally, so does nitric oxide and even carbon monoxide, in the right amounts). I anticipate that the gut-*gas*-brain connection will become one of the most important breakthroughs in the fight against our neurodegenerative disease epidemic. Odd as it may sound, to some extent you *want* your brain to be "full of hot air."

Sadly, many people are consuming foods that actively prevent their gut bugs from producing these brain-protecting compounds. If you've ever wondered why a high-sugar diet is bad for your brain, it's partly because it reduces your gut biome's population of lactobacilli, those anti-inflammatory bugs that help make protective short-chain fatty acids.[27] Even worse, in conjunction with high levels of saturated fat, sugar can start to cause its memory-impairing damage after only a few days—regardless of whether or not you are overweight. Sugar and high levels of saturated fat are your brain's worst enemies. They cause you to store fat around your midsection (to fuel the inflammatory war that's going on around a leaky gut). If you're familiar with my previous work, you may recall my saying "Fat in your gut; you're out of luck!" I really mean that: An uptick of fat in your gut is directly connected to "cognitive aging"—and you don't need to be a scientist to know you want to avoid that.[28]

Once the fire of inflammation spreads from your gut to your brain, it is a sign that a wildfire is already burning in your body. And like a wildfire, it's imperative to get a handle on the spread sooner rather than later—before the widespread damage is done and all your health and energy protecting resources are exhausted.

Pruning Gone Wild

When microglial pruning is left unchecked, over time it can spin out of control. In an effort to protect the neuron at all costs, the unintended consequence is a starved, dying neuron. That's how pruning can lead to dementia, Alzheimer's and Parkinson's. (The Lewy body, made notorious by Robin Williams's battle with Lewy body disease, is a dead neuron surrounded by microglia, a pathologic finding seen in the brain and gut neurons in Parkinson's patients.) Moreover, about 30 percent of the population has a gene that makes them more susceptible to neuroinflammation; it's called the APOE4 gene (also known as the Alzheimer's gene). It tells the microglia to incite an inflammatory state anytime they sense impending danger, and consequently in their overenthusiasm, they vastly overproduce nitric oxide,[29] further increasing neuroinflammation.

If you have the APOE4 gene, you have less wiggle room in your diet than those who don't. As Dr. Bredesen and I agree, a program that limits lectins, promotes postbiotic-making foods, and shortens your eating window as a way to promote mitochondrial flexibility (which is the foundation of the Energy Paradox Program) can help protect you from cognitive decline.

Acute Stress on the Brain

If you've ever experienced a period of sustained, seemingly unending, heightened stress, you probably know how tiring it can be. All you want to do is take a nap, pour yourself a glass of wine, or simply shut down and hide. You might even have moments of feeling gripped or paralyzed with shock. In fact, you likely experienced something like this during the global COVID-19 pandemic. For so many people facing the stress and anxiety of the pandemic, bedtime couldn't come soon enough (though, ironically, you may also have had trouble sleeping). None of this exhaustion is imagined. Whether high stress is acute and shocking or chronic and unrelenting, it will stealthily contribute to leaky gut and inflammation that, in turn, can steal your energy reserves and, over time, compound the neuroinflammation that's simultaneously inflaming and starving your brain.

I see a phenomenon in my practice where some patients with autoimmune disease can point to a highly stressful event as the onset of their condition. (It's typically women who do this; partly because they're more connected to their bodies, and partly because as we now understand, women are more susceptible to physical effects of stress than men.) I'm empathetic but never surprised, because acute stress can literally damage the gut wall cells, starting the downward slide to leaky gut and inflammation. It's an evolutionary trait: Under emergency conditions, your sympathetic nerves divert blood flow away from your digestive system to fuel your muscles into action. (The old "fight-or-flee a saber-toothed tiger" scenario.) Depriving cells of enough oxygen for even a few minutes (four, to be exact) can cause them to die—technically it's called *hypoxia*. It prunes your roots on what should be a flourishing intestinal wall—and as you know, "pruned roots" in your gut are as bad for your energy and clarity as "pruned neurons" in your brain.

I'm sorry to say that's not all: To make matters worse, the "assault" of stress switches on the inflammatory immune cells that live in your gut while also changing the composition of your gut microbiome in favor of the bugs that erode your gut wall.[30] And when your gut wall becomes more permeable, it's less able to resist pathogenic bacteria. Perhaps it becomes clearer now how a genuinely shocking event (an accident, a death, divorce, or un-expected loss, or a global pandemic) can trigger such ill health; it starts by taking a huge toll on the permeability of the gut wall, un-leashing inflammation that then sends signals to the microglia in your brain to prepare for the worst. The stress leads to confusion, dullness, and a slower, starved brain—which in turn begets more stress, because you start to fear something is really wrong. Making matters worse, your imbalanced biome is now less able to help you generate the neurotransmitters that help you feel focused and alert (like norepinephrine),[31] or that help you feel a sense of ease and calm (like GABA, which calms an overactive nervous system) and all-around well-being (serotonin and the precursors to serotonin like tryptophan and 5-HTP). Without the right neurotransmitters present, your already overwhelmed brain will take a further hit and your mood and cognition will suffer.

If you've ever endured an extremely stressful situation (and who hasn't?), you know that in the moment, you often feel a yearning for comfort foods that "dull the pain" by giving you a quick hit of sugar and perhaps serotonin, which rapidly wears off, requiring you to get another and then another fake high of pleasure: the exact high-sugar, high-fat foods that compound the problem by starving your gut buddies of the fuel they need (and feeding the ones you don't want around). Of course, these foods also overwhelm your mito-chondrial energy factories, making you feel tired and listless. And when you're sluggish you're less prone to get the exercise your mi-tochondria need to function, further draining your energy while also robbing you of your natural abundance of alertness-promoting neurotransmitters. Bam! Now you're stressed, exhausted, unmo-tivated, and can't see the way out. But that's why you're here: In the Energy Paradox Program, you'll lift your way out of this funk by adding some quick exercises (what I call "snacks") into your pro-gram that will turn *on* your energy factories, not slow them down.

Just as the microbiota-gut-brain axis is bidirectional, so is stress and leaky-gut-induced inflammation. A stressed gut can contribute to mental stress and unease . . . which can then broadcast unease back *down* to the gut via the vagus nerve and the cycle continues. This gives new perspective to why, if you're chronically tired, managing your stress is not an optional activity. You have to actively seize it by the throat (so to speak) and find a way that works for you to get a handle on it.

As I like to remind my patients, life and stress aren't things that happen *to* you. Events happen, sometimes challenging ones, and your body either tips into a dysfunctional stress response or, if you catch it happening, you can take control and find ways to dissipate it. Perhaps you were taught that the fight-or-flight reflex is entirely unconscious—your body, spurred by the ancient "reptilian" part of your brain, reflexively surges with stress hormones at that fabled saber-toothed tiger (or parking cop, or mean boss). However, this long-standing theory is no longer considered accurate; science is now showing how your *conscious* thoughts—the ones you choose to have—can either activate your stress hormone network and, by association, your gut, or calm it all down. In Part II, we will look at how to harness the power of your mind to reduce and manage stress while you are restoring the gut-brain axis back to normal.

The Insulin-Resistant Brain

In addition to the quiet, unrecognized fire of neuroinflammation, the average modern brain also tends to get bogged down as a result of the mitochondrial logjam we discussed in Chapter 4. If your mitochondria are overworked and overwhelmed, you can bet you're going to feel the same way.

From my experience in working with patients who've lost (and then thankfully regained) their mental sharpness, I can attest that when your get-up-and-go has gone missing, and when you find yourself getting more forgetful, it's likely that you are losing insulin sensitivity and metabolic flexibility in the brain. Just like other cells in your body protect themselves by becoming resistant to insulin's actions, your neurons become starved of glucose because insulin is being blocked by ceramides,[32] as we discussed previously. And without fuel for the mitochondria to make energy, your neurons cannot work well, and so how can you think clearly? If you have an elevated fasting insulin level of 9 uIU/ml or above, I can assure you that your entire body, including your brain, is insulin resistant. This means that you've lost your ability to make free fatty acids and ketones from your stored fat to use as the alternative fuel in your mitochondria; in short, you have no metabolic flexibility. Sadly, the typical Western diet has created a scenario in which ceramide-induced insulin resistance is occurring in the brain, starving it of energy, driving up inflammation, and blocking mitochondrial function.[33] Talk about a hit in the head!

Insulin, in low amounts of course, is needed to communicate with the receptors on your neurons, just like other cells. There's a "sweet spot" of insulin in your bloodstream that supports your overall health by balancing hunger hormones and regulating appetite, helping to reduce neuroinflammation, helping your cognition to stay sharp. But as the receptors for insulin become more insulated in your body, the same phenomenon is taking place in your neurons. You may not have heard the term type 3 diabetes or diabetes of the brain *yet* (likely you've heard of type 1 and type 2 diabetes), but given the way the research is going, this will soon become a common diagnosis. Type 3 diabetes refers to a full spectrum of neurological decline, from mild cognitive impairment all the way to full-blown dementia, which is almost always predicated on insulin resistance in the brain.[34] As I shared in the last chapter, it's not really accurate to use the term *prediabetes*—if you are diagnosed as prediabetic, you are already insulin resistant. Similarly, I don't want to downplay a "little bit" of diabetes of the brain—it is that slippery a slope.

There are ways to ensure your brain retains (or restores) its innate sensitivity to insulin, meaning it can hear the doorbell ring of insulin and open the door to fuel and gain its neuroprotective effects. We will talk about these strategies in detail in Part II, but they are based on the following four goals:

1. Reducing the workload on the mitochondria through carefully timed eating.

2. Removing the foods that rush sugars into your system (which cue the pancreas to make more insulin, in turn creating insulin-resistant cells).

3. Adding in foods like walnuts, olive oil, and sesame oil that actually inhibit ceramide production.[35]

4. Feeding your gut buddies, which help to maintain insulin sensitivity through the compounds they make.[36]

A neuron has the capacity to grow new dendrites just like a plant grows roots and shoots. These new dendrites give you the ability to keep making new connections between neurons that help you stay sharp and clear, with a well-preserved memory too. But it can't do that without energy—a starved neuron is not going to grow new shoots. Which means all the sudoku and crossword puzzles in the world can't compensate. If you want a clear, alert brain today and for all the tomorrows that follow, you want to *help* your brain access energy. And that starts with how and what you feed it.

ENERGY MYTH #5: My Overgrowth of Candida Is Tiring Me Out

If I had a nickel for every time I've heard this one. It seems to be a trend: blaming chronic fatigue on a fungus. But candida overgrowth is not, in my experience, the real source of energy drains. Candida is a normal yeast in everyone, one of many that reside in your gut. Candida is not harmful in and of itself; it becomes a problem when it outcompetes the other guys for food and starts growing too fast, creating a condition called *candidiasis*. This imbalance can happen after a course of antibiotics that wipe out your gut buddies or as a result of eating a high-sugar diet, as sugar essentially fuels the reproduction of candida. (Remember, we make beer and wine by giving yeasts sugar, in particular fructose, to eat.)

Candidiasis has become, in my opinion, an overdiagnosed condition, and in reality, resolving a fungal overgrowth is not that complicated. I've had patients tell me they're following strict anti-candida diets along with taking supplements or even antifungal medications to "kill the candida." My advice is to take a look at your diet and remove the simple sugars (including the fructose in fruits) and refined grains as well as the saturated fats that preferentially feed the less-helpful bugs in your biome. When you take the bad things out and put the right things in, the gut will take care of rebalancing itself over time. The point is not to kill off candida completely. You don't want that, because mysterious as their purpose may be, all bugs bring something to the table. For example, your gut naturally contains gluten-eating bacteria—bugs that feast on gluten and break down that protein for you, rendering it less harmful. When you go 100 percent gluten-free, you can actually hurt yourself by starving out those helpful bugs, so that any occasional bite of gluten becomes intolerable. Your inborn defense system against the odd gluten that sneaks into your diet (and it does, believe me) is gone. This is why I advocate a natural rebalancing of the ecosystem when possible, rather than attempting to decimate any one of its members. This reminds me of the mistake of removing wolves from Yellowstone Park, which resulted in a massive overgrowth of elk and a decimation of the entire ecosystem. Was the answer to kill off the elk? Of course not; just put the wolves back and within a few years, the normal balance returned.

CHAPTER 6

IT'S ALL ABOUT TIMING
(AND GOOD CHOICES)

As you'll recall from the beginning of the book, I've devised a simple equation to help explain how human energy is created: $E = M^2C^2$. We've now fully explored the first half of this equation—the two Ms of microbiome and mitochondria. We know that energy is dependent on a robust and diverse community of gut buddies as well as high-functioning mitochondria. So now let's turn to the last piece of the puzzle, those Cs. These are the most actionable parts of the equation, the ones that can help you recover your get-up-and-go and start feeling like yourself again faster than you may think.

But I have to be honest: This part of the journey is going to be a little uncomfortable.

"Uncomfortable?" I hear you asking. "I want more energy, not discomfort, Dr. G." Now, I get it; as humans, we intrinsically dislike even the thought of experiencing something that challenges us; we gravitate toward what is familiar and thus "safe." But in this instance, what is familiar is far from safe—it's the culprit behind our lethargy and malaise. Sometimes it's good to push through a little discomfort.

Let me give you a personal example. When I was younger, I had to walk a mile to and from school (in all kinds of weather, if that meant in rain, through a foot of snow, blah, blah, blah); I mowed the lawn with a push mower; I shoveled snow with a shovel; I raked leaves with a rake; I opened and closed garage doors by hand (imagine!); and even got up to walk to the TV to change the channel. You get the picture—that was back in "the old days"; but as I grew up and became an adult, I didn't do much of that anymore. Why? Because, well, it's work, it's time-consuming, it's a pain in the neck, and it's just plain easier and more comfortable to use the marvelous inventions that make it possible to avoid backbreaking chores. Unfortunately, because of this, I drifted too far from what my cells and mitochondria required to stay fit—the naturally challenging conditions that would force them to work their hardest. Little by little, I became more sedentary, more comfortable, increasingly fatigued—and less healthy.

Cut to my life about twenty years ago. If you have read my previous books, you may remember my life was jolted by meeting a patient whom I called "Big Ed." Big Ed had reversed his severe inoperable coronary artery disease by a change in diet that involved completely banishing inflammatory lectins and taking supplements. Not only that, but he restored his metabolic flexibility, regained his insulin sensitivity and mental clarity, and reclaimed the energy he'd had as a younger man. I was, quite frankly, in awe of his dramatic turnaround.

After experimenting on myself (by following my Yale University dietary thesis on the early human diet) and losing seventy pounds in the process, I started my Centers for Restorative Medicine to teach patients how to reverse heart disease, diabetes, and subsequently autoimmune diseases with food, supplements, and one more thing that I came to value highly: changes to the timing of their meals. As this transition to a new pattern of eating would often meet with some resistance, I would tell my patients to "embrace their hunger." And perhaps oddly enough, within days, their hunger would leave and never return again.

For my part, six months out of the year (from January to June), I restrict my eating window during the week to two hours a day, so that twenty-two out of every twenty-four hours I am not eating, with time off during the weekends for "good behavior." I dub this "Enjoy One Meal a Day" or EOMAD. (Just as a fun aside, some of my patients call it "Gundry's One Meal a Day," or, you guessed it: GOMAD!) These months correspond to the times of the year when, in nature, less food would generally be available. (Let's be clear, even in the jungle, there are circadian rhythms of food availability depending on the season. In winter and spring, less food; summer and fall, more food.) The other six months—corresponding to more plentiful food in summer and fall—I increase my eating window to six or eight hours, and do not eat for sixteen to eighteen hours, to balance out my own seasonal circadian rhythms. The practice of limiting the time you consume calories is usually called time-restricted eating, and long before it became fashionable, or even written about, I was practicing it and writing about it, with my first book way back in 2006. I just finished my eighteenth year of this practice and I haven't "gone mad." In fact, just the opposite. But don't panic, unless you want to try EOMAD, as a turbo charged version of the Energy Paradox Program, none of you need to GOMAD.

So, what did I know way back then that has only recently been documented so well? Decades ago I became fascinated with the idea of *hormesis*, or beneficial stress. To understand why going *without* food for longer than you might initially choose can actually increase your energy levels tremendously, it's important to understand why a touch of discomfort makes you stronger.

In geeky terms, hormesis is known as the *biphasic dose response*. It is a biological law that describes how bodily systems can be activated or "turned on" by low doses of any physical insult, stressor, or chemical substance—even if those very same things are toxic in large doses.

I prefer a snappier description of this natural law, stated by Nietzsche (and decades later sung by my pal Kelly Clarkson): "What doesn't kill you makes you stronger." Plants illustrate this principle quite nicely. Plants that grow in conditions of mild but persistent stress don't necessarily wither or fail as might be expected. In fact, they start producing higher amounts of *xenohormetic* (say that three times in a row!) molecules—protective compounds like resveratrol in grapes, or melatonin that we mentioned earlier, that in turn boost their health, and consequently our health, when we consume them. Hormesis essentially says to any living thing, any cell, any mitochondria, and any gene: Hard times are coming, we need to get more resilient, stronger, fitter, and able to survive. One of my friends and colleagues, renowned Harvard longevity expert Dr. David Sinclair, calls this level of mild stress on the system "*a state of perceived adversity.*" Not challenging enough to actually be damaging, but enough to *give your cells the impression that times are going to be tough.* This is such an important, if counterintuitive, concept for regaining your energy that I want to reiterate it: Even if you are fatigued, challenging your body is beneficial. It's about tricking your biology in a sense, sending it environmental signals that flip the switch on its preprogrammed response to adversity. And using a controlled eating timetable is one way to achieve this.

We're going to take it easy here, though: I'm going to ask you to progressively extend the natural period of the day (and night) when you don't eat. Yes, the time you are not eating is called fasting, but I'm referring to a very specific form of fasting here—time-controlled eating—which is subtly, but importantly, different from time-restricted eating. And let's be clear about this: You will not need to eat less food or count calories. I just want to control when you eat those calories.

Discomfort: A Little Dab'll Do Ya

Our bodies are not only designed for challenge, they are built to thrive with just the right amount of perceived adversity. So all this modern dodging of discomfort has thrown us for a loop. As much as we may dislike it, we *need* moderate levels of biological and environmental stressors. For example, a plethora of recent studies about the benefits of fasting, as well as *cryotherapy* (the use of cold), and even heat/sauna therapy—all things that can make us uncomfortable but are, in a sense, the driving forces of nature—have shown that each of these interventions provide real health benefits. When exposed to the mild stresses of temporary lack of food or to extremes of cold and heat, cells engage in coordinated *adaptive measures* that stimulate them to clean up, repair, and re-store themselves while calming down any inflammation. Fasting alone can lead to increased expression of antioxidant defenses, DNA repair, protein quality control, mitochondrial biogenesis and autophagy, and downregulation of inflammation.[1]

Here's the good news: I'm not going to ask you to stop eating (whew!). I'm just going to ask you to *time your eating* better. And that's C^2 in the energy equation. I call it *chrono consumption*, because it is about coordinating both the timing of *when* you are going to eat and *what* you are going to consume during those eating windows. It's a doable way of consuming your calories in a controlled fashion that will protect and boost your mitochondrial function so that you are more efficient at making energy. It also improves the diversity and abundance of the good guys in your microbiome,[2] and changes their circadian rhythm as well.[3] Besides resetting the microbiome clocks, chrono consumption also helps to reset the circadian clock that exists in every one of your cells and helps to upregulate many of the genes that keep you vital, peppy, and fit. As paradoxical as it sounds, limiting access to energy sources (food) to a limited time period, and going without food for longer periods of time, actually increases your overall energy. Put simply, chrono consumption will regulate what fuels you give your mitochondria and how much time they spend doing the work of making energy for you—freeing up more energy for you to do all the things you want to do!

A Lexicon of Fasting

Before we dive into what I consider the best of the best of fasting, which we'll use in the Energy Paradox Program, let's take a minute to define our terms.

As many of you likely know, fasting simply refers to the practice of forgoing food for a certain amount of time. Where *feeding* is a state of building and growing (helping to build tissues and grow muscles), fasting can be and should be a repair state, when protective mechanisms kick in and the cellular energy system gets time to reprogram itself, scanning for errors and fixing glitches. Your design needs time for both and it needs significant time without processing food for energy to switch over into "fasting physiology." As I've written previously, while your health is predicated on what you eat, your weight, metabolism, gut biome, heart health, inflammation, sleep, and, most important, energy production are equally (or more) influenced by *when* you eat. In particular, these factors are influenced by whether you leave enough time between feedings for your body to enter its much-needed fasted state.[4]

However, *fasting* is an umbrella term—and not every type of fasting is the same. The terms *intermittent fasting* and *time-restricted eating* (or feeding) are often used interchangeably by the general public, but in the nutritional research community, intermittent fasting has a more specific definition, referring to a water-only or very-low-calorie period lasting about twenty-four hours and followed by a normal feeding period of one to two days. Also included in this definition is the so-called 5:2 diet, first popularized in 2012, where you eat about 600 calories two days a week and eat "normally" the other days; as well as *alternate day fasting*, where you eat one day, then skip the next, and so on (this diet is very popular in mice studies but pretty much a failure in human trials due to compliance issues).[5] There is also a longer form of intermittent fasting popularized by my friend and colleague Dr. Jason Fung, where you generally have nothing but water and perhaps electrolytes for at least seventy-two hours.

Another form of fasting is the practice of calorie restriction with optimal nutrition, the so-called CRON diet (shortened to CR in most studies), popularized by the late Dr. Roy Walford, which reduces calorie intake on a daily basis by about 25 to 30 percent from "normal." This type of restriction also triggers the state of *fasting physiology*, and it is, as of yet, the only proven way to maximally extend the life span of all animals tested except for rhesus monkeys (we will get to that study shortly). Finally, there is the fasting mimicking diet, created by my friend Dr. Valter Longo at USC (Dr. Walford's protégé!), in which you eat an 800 to 1100 calorie vegan diet for five days in a row, once a month. This approach has been shown to mimic most of the effects of a three- to five-day water fast or a monthlong 30 percent calorie restriction.

As beneficial as all these methods are for weight loss and possibly longevity, I believe they pale in comparison to a program that combines the many benefits of time-restricted eating while priming the pump, so to speak, with the first meal of the day being composed primarily of one fuel type, whether it be carbs, proteins, or fats. Remember the "mono" diets we discussed in Chapter 4, which (seemingly preposterously) restrict intake to one type of food? While I don't recommend a nutritional protocol of eating only one type of food for months or years on end, those diets *are* effective because they eliminate the mitochondrial traffic jam that occurs when you consume too many different fuel sources at once. That's why the C^2 part of my program takes the best of fasting and mono approaches, combining time-restricted eating with one mono meal. Now, you may be thinking, where's the evidence to back up this crazy hybrid eating plan? Well, I'm glad you asked.

For years, longevity researchers debated over two competing studies on how caloric restriction impacted longevity in rhesus monkeys. One was conducted by the NIH's National Institute on Aging (NIA) and the other was conducted at the University of Wisconsin (UW). Both studies spanned over thirty years, comparing the health span (the absence of age-related diseases) as well as the life span between a group of rhesus monkeys that were put on a calorie-restricted diet (a 30 percent reduction) and a control group of monkeys that were not. While both caloric restriction groups had vastly improved health spans compared to normally fed monkeys, only the UW study showed evidence of increased longevity. I and others have postulated that although both groups were given the same number of limited calories, the actual makeup of the calories eaten were wildly different, with the UW monkeys getting a relatively high-sucrose (that's good old table sugar, half glucose and half fructose) and high-fat diet, while the NIH group was given a diet that was lower in sugar and fat, but had more fiber and protein. But just to be clear, both groups got 60 percent of their calories from carbs. Since only the UW group showed improved longevity, I and other longevity researchers argued that it was because of the lower protein content in that group's diet. But the debate raged on.

Enter Dr. Rafael de Cabo, also at the NIH, to settle the score in 2018.[6] He took approximately 300 mice (okay sticklers, 292 to be exact) and separated them into six groups. Three groups ate the UW higher-sucrose, higher-fat, lower-protein diet, while the other three groups ate the NIA lower-sucrose, lower-fat, higher-protein diet. To make things interesting, one set of mice in each diet got access to their food twenty-four hours a day; one set in each group were calorie restricted to 30 percent fewer calories and fed once a day starting at 3 p.m., so they had a shorter eating window. The final two sets got the full caloric amount, but their food was put out at 3 p.m. as well, to control whether the *timing* of eating was actually why calorie-restricted animals lived longer. (I'll call these the "time-restricted eating" mice.) Why is that so important for you and me to understand in regard to this book? Think of it this way: If you get 30 percent less food every day, and it arrives all at once as your daily ration, guess how fast it will be eaten? So, sure enough, the calorie-restricted guys gobbled up their chow quickly (the high-sucrose and high-fat group ate quickest! No surprise there, it was gone in an hour); the twenty-four-hour groups kind of nibbled all day and night, sadly much like we do (but mice eat mostly at night); while the "time-restricted eating" mice finished their food in nine to twelve hours and fasted for the rest (that's a really long time for a mouse to not eat, by the way).

So what to make of all of this? We have the all-day slow munchers, the binge calorie-restricted eaters, and the full-calorie but time-restricted eating guys. Can you guess which group fared best? Well, only two of the groups showed evidence of metabolic flexibility, and it wasn't the all-day eaters, it was the ones whose diets allowed for plenty of time without food. Now, shockingly, it didn't matter whether they were the high-sucrose group or the high-fat group. And it didn't matter if they were calorie restricted or got full calories, as long as the eating window was condensed. Both sets of mice developed metabolic flexibility, with mitochondria that could switch easily between fuels. But the mice who nibbled around the clock (with time off for sleeping) had no mitochondrial flexibility. They were stuck.

Finally, here's the longevity punchline: The calorie-restricted guys lived nearly 30 percent longer than the twenty-four-hour eaters (no surprise here), but interestingly, the makeup of their diet made no difference at all. Okay, great, close the book, drop your calories every day by 30 percent, and live forever. But, if you really stopped reading now, you'd miss the bigger point. Remember, these calorie-restricted mice ate all their meager allotment of food rapidly and were *fasting for most of the twenty-four hours.* And the time-restricted mice that didn't have to calorie restrict, but still had lengthy fasting periods? They lived 11 percent longer than the all-day eaters. In human terms, that would translate into improving the life span by ten years and, more important, improving our overall health span. It was the time period when they weren't eating, more than the composition of the diet, that had the most significant impact.

Want some human proof of a similar effect? A recent Italian study showed that a regimen of time-restricted eating, particularly when combined with regular exercise, results in many long-term adaptations that improve mental and physical performance and protect against disease.[7] In this study, two groups of healthy athletes ate the same calorically controlled diet. One group of participants ate three regular meals at 8 a.m., 1 p.m., and 8 p.m. (finishing at 9 p.m., a thirteen-hour eating window), and the other group ate the same meals at 1 p.m., 4 p.m., and 8 p.m. (an eight-hour window). The eight-hour eating window (which is what you will work up to slowly in the Energy Paradox Program) resulted in both fat loss and muscle mass growth, while simultaneously lowering insulin-like growth factor (IGF-1), which drives the aging process. The twelve-hour eaters had no such benefits, including no weight loss, despite eating the exact same number of calories. Put another nail in the coffin of "calories in = calories out." The time-controlled eating worked by challenging organ systems just enough to become more resilient, stronger, and healthier.

The big idea here is not that fasting has a positive effect—we've known that for some time—but rather, it's not what you eat that matters most, but when and for how long you eat it that's important to how well your metabolism and energy system work. One last proviso, before you decide to eat M&M's as your only meal of the day to live forever: Obviously, all the mice in the longevity study did die; but interestingly, the high-sucrose, high-fat diet mice died more often from liver cancer than any other cause; and (maybe the best news) all the time-restricted groups had significantly less amyloid (the plaques found in Alzheimer's and dementia patients' brains) in their tissues than the twenty-four-hour eating guys. So not only was time-controlled eating proven to benefit energy production and enhance life span—it also offered neuroprotective effects.

Could Everything You Thought You Knew about Nutrition Be Wrong?

Okay great, Dr. G, so monkeys and mice benefit from time-controlled eating. What does that mean for us? Well, for one thing, it throws conventional wisdom on its head. Think about it. Contrast these studies, and hundreds of others like them,[8,9] with the long-standing nutritional mainstay of "three square meals plus two snacks a day," starting with a big breakfast upon rising and ending with a significant dinner (and dessert) close to bedtime. A host of forces (including the breakfast cereal industry, the dairy industry, and the citrus industry) have conspired to make us believe that of these, breakfast is our most important meal. I say—and forgive my directness—that this is ludicrous. From an evolutionary point of view, this concept fails to hold water. Your ancestors would have found the idea of making time for breakfast—followed by a sizable lunch and a bigger dinner in the fourteen hours that followed—very peculiar indeed. In fact, your whole hormonal operating system is designed as if breakfast wasn't going to happen.[10]

In the early morning hours, your adrenal glands start secreting more cortisol and epinephrine (adrenaline) into your bloodstream, causing your liver to make more glucose available, even after an overnight fast (i.e., hours with no food in your system). Interesting, huh? It's as if our bodies were designed to be "up and at 'em" regardless of whether or not we happened to have access to food. Remember, your ancestors did not crawl out of their caves at sunrise and plop some eggs in a frying pan or pour a bowl of cereal. There were no food storage systems; once they tracked down or foraged some food, they ate most of it pretty much immediately.

Then there's this bad advice: Consume small meals throughout the day to ensure your blood sugar stays "stable" and so your energy doesn't "crash." (Spoiler alert: If your energy levels are rising and crashing throughout the day without injections of food, that's a call to take a look under the metabolic hood!) Here's the problem. Remember the fate of the poor mice that followed that dietary advice? They had no metabolic flexibility; they could not make the switch to burning fat as a fuel when sugars ran out. They were stuck being able to only burn sugar to make energy. They had the shortest life span and no metabolic flexibility, the exact opposite of what you and I are looking for. As you will soon learn, the Energy Paradox Program will support your energy as you make the transition. So, no, your blood sugar will not crash at first, like other programs; furthermore, fasting creates increased insulin sensitivity, which will actually stabilize blood sugar in the long run—allowing you to get off the roller coaster entirely.

So, it's time to reconsider these preconceptions of how we fuel our bodies. For example, consider those high-protein energy bars and shakes that are all the rage these days. Do they help your body gear up for a workout as promised? Hardly. For one thing, digestion is energy-expensive and requires huge amounts of blood flowing to your intestines to get the job done. If it's going there to digest your meal or snack, not much blood flow is left for your muscles.[11] In fact, when it comes to what to eat before a workout, research demonstrates that athletes actually perform better in a fasted state.[12] Far from flailing when a meal is slightly postponed, we actually perform closer to optimal on an empty stomach. Think of your very ancient human ancestors—the ones living without the fridge and pantry stocked full of vittles. If they hadn't eaten for a baker's dozen of hours, perhaps days, they'd need *more* clarity, focus, and sprint power than normal in order to make sure they captured some juicy fish or game at the very next opportunity! Or had the strength to walk ten to twenty miles in search of edible food.[13] Because for the body, the natural rhythm is feast . . . and then famine—or at least a period of waiting for the next opportunity to eat. Your body expects there to be a fluctuation between the two states: feed, then fast, then feed, then fast. Swinging between these extremes programs the clocks in your cells that help keep your metabolism on track and your inflammation in check.

Time-Controlled Eating Resets Your Body Clocks

As you have now read, activities in your body respond to daily fluctuations in your environment, which, to state it simply, keep your body on a schedule. We usually talk about light as the primary cue for setting this schedule: Changes between light and dark give the master circadian clock in your body, the suprachiasmatic nucleus (SCN), data that signals hormones to activate or deactivate genes for almost every process you can think of, from short-term energy production to long-term resistance and disease. Like a plant, you are designed to live in sync with the cycles of the sun and the rhythm of the natural world. Perhaps you have experienced how when you work late or all-night hours, or cross time zones regularly, your weight, mood, and many other functions suffer alongside your energy. The regular schedule of daylight to darkness that your body expects has gotten topsy-turvy, and hormones driving sleep, metabolism, and anti-inflammation have gotten all mixed up. But what has only recently been discovered is how much your eating patterns also signal the clocks in your body to activate important pathways for your metabolism, energy, and overall health.

In addition to the SCN, all the cells in your body have their own clocks (called peripheral clocks), and it turns out they are especially attuned to the fluctuations of feeding and fasting.[14] Even your microbiome has a circadian clock. All these various clocks expect a full belly part of the day, and an empty one—a fasted state—for much of the rest of the day. And when you don't give them the fasted part because you are digesting and processing food for too many hours, your clocks get the "wrong time" and don't turn on all the activities your energy system needs to work its best.[15]

For most of our evolution, we ate according to a predictable schedule, timed to sunlight. No breakfast, as I mentioned, and likely no eating after dark. (And, if we did eat after dark, we would have been exposed to red and orange light from a fire, not blue light like we are now.) Longer periods of eating during summer (more light for hunting and gathering and eating) and shorter periods during winter. Our circadian clocks developed in line with this natural rhythm; during certain periods of the day our genes direct a lot of resources to the ATP production line, while other periods of the day are allocated for repair time. When we eat according to this natural rhythm, our bodies can perform optimally.

Let me give you an example of how this plays out in today's world: Those who follow the religion of Islam observe the month of Ramadan, during which practitioners abstain from food and drink from dawn to dusk, eating one meal to "break the fast" after sunset, sleeping, then waking to another meal before sunrise as the lead in to dawn prayer. Once a year, this ritual is practiced every day for thirty days.

Studies on groups of Muslims (all volunteers) have revealed that this practice of time-controlled eating during Ramadan had significant benefits on participants' short- and long-term health.[16,17] Genes that encode for cancer (*oncogenes*) were suppressed, while protective protein-making genes were switched *on*. Researchers found that many of the proteins that help regulate insulin, metabolize sugars and fats properly (thus promote more efficient energy making), and protect against neuron damage were all given a boost. Even better, there was an elevation in proteins that help mitochondria repair themselves, as well as those that quell both immune-driven inflammation and other systemic sources of inflammation. Thus, just by changing eating patterns—and "resetting" the circadian clocks that tend to get scrambled by our modern lifestyle—the study participants switched on a host of health-promoting benefits, many of which are energy boosters.

Today most of us live a lifestyle that looks nothing like the fasting of Ramadan, but instead reminds me of the classic TV game show *Beat the Clock*. Unfortunately, our epidemic of fatigue and modern diseases is showing us that the clock cannot be beat. Another study involving human volunteers, carried out by circadian researcher Dr. Satchin Panda at the Salk Institute, showed that reducing your "feeding" time (whether you're a mouse or a human being) to ten hours—leaving fourteen hours of non-eating—conferred huge benefits over eating and digesting for fifteen hours and fasting for nine or fewer hours. Dr. Panda found that even when slightly overweight people reduced their eating window to ten hours, they reset their cellular clocks and lost weight, were much more energetic, slept better, had improved moods and sharper thinking—all over the course of just a few months.[18]

If you're wondering how changing your eating schedule could lead to benefits like improved mood and cognition, it's because fasting offers your brain a good kind of challenge—hormesis—which it responds to meet by activating stress-response pathways that help your brain cope with stress and resist disease. (This holds true even if you have genes that predispose you to neuro-degenerative diseases: Fasting protects the neurons in mice with engineered genes for Parkinson's and Alzheimer's diseases, allowing them to perform better in mazes when testing learning and memory.)[19] Remember, in a fasted state your brain can get sharper and clearer because your brain perceives that it had better help you track down some food, stat! If you don't get into the game or catch some game, it's curtains.

Your Mitochondria Can Tell the Time

Your circadian rhythm is so impactful, it even governs how much energy you make and when you make it. A University of Basel study demonstrated for the first time exactly how cellular energy metabolism also follows the rhythm of the circadian clock—something that hitherto had been a little mysterious.[20] It has to do with the rhythms of what's called the *mitochondrial fission-fusion cycle*—an innate feature of mitochondria that allows them to fuse together in connected networks, and then divide. The mitochondrial network interacts with the circadian clocks via a protein called *DRP1*. This rhythm is integral to determining how much energy the mitochondria can supply and when. The time of day thus influences the cell's energy capacity—makes sense, right?—but conversely, if the circadian clock is out of whack, it causes the mitochondrial network to lose its rhythm and make less energy in the cells. Just another reason why late nights scrolling through social media can make you feel so sluggish the next day. It's not only all that junk light that's sent your melatonin levels on a downslide; you've literally compromised your cellular energy production by confusing your body clocks.

Ketones: A Fuel Source that Signals Repair

In Chapter 4, I described how your body, under ideal circumstances, switches between fuel sources, or "fluctuates" on a schedule. If you remember, glucose and fatty acids are the main sources of fuel for mitochondria to produce ATP. After meals, glucose is used for energy production; any excess is converted to glycogen (the storage form of glucose), and if even more is left over, it is converted to fat and stored in adipose (fat) tissue. Normally, starting about ten hours after a meal, all that glucose gets used up, including the stored glycogen in cells. Sensing the tanks are empty, your cells cry, *Glucose stores are gone! We need other fuel!* That call for energy triggers stored fat to be released from fat cells by hormone-sensitive lipase activation (now no longer suppressed by insulin) to get broken down to free fatty acids and glycerol, which can circulate freely into all cells (except the brain), enter the mitochondrial assembly line, and be used to produce ATP. As more time passes after your last meal, twelve hours or so now, some of those fatty acids are transported to the liver, where they get converted into the ketones. Just to review, free fatty acids can't get into the brain easily or quickly—so ketones become your brain mitochondria's primary fuel source during a fasted state. When your mitochondria successfully "switch" energy sources in this way, it helps build your metabolic flexibility—and the more you do it (by increasing time between meals), the more metabolically flexible, and more insulin sensitive, you become. Greater metabolic flexibility allows you to process a variety of fuels efficiently. In other words: It's less likely for your favorite carbs to show up later as belly fat. Now that's what I'm takin' about! It's liberating!

You also start to reap the protective benefits of the fasted physiology. Ketones are powerful signaling molecules that tell your mitochondria, cells, and organs to reboot, rejuvenate, and energize themselves.[21] The levels of ketone bodies in the blood tend to be very low when you are fed, but by twelve hours after eating, they are rising nicely (and by twenty-four hours of going food free, they are significant).[22] Let's be certain you see the connection: Your cells, guided by their circadian clock, expect there to be an oscillation between fuel sources, depending on whether you are fed or fasted. When you leave *at least* twelve hours between meals, you shift into a state in which free fatty acids and ketones come to the fore. It's these guys that signal your cells and mitochondria that times are likely to be tough and not much food is available (at least as far as they can tell) so you better make sure all systems are in peak condition. Cellular efficiency increases and mitochondrial protection and repair processes switch on, including antioxidant defenses against overproduced and damaging ROSs. (The technical term for this is *mitohormesis*.) Mitogenesis—mitochondrial replication—also gets turned on, as does the cellular cleanup system called *autophagy*, which removes damaged molecules and recycles their components, thereby reducing inflammation. Unbeknownst to you, fasting also helps your mitochondria increase the production of hydrogen sulfide,[23] almost like an alternative fuel source that is especially helpful if your ATP production is impaired[24]—exactly the extra support we are looking for! Hydrogen sulfide literally makes mitochondria stronger.[25,26]

This cellular cascade of effects has huge benefits for you and your energy. You've not only restored your metabolic flexibility and energy efficiency by training your cells to use fatty acids for fuel, you're also benefiting from the ketones signaling your cellular energy system to do the maintenance work it needs to function well. It's as if the road crew got the signal that freeways are clear of vehicles and they can go patch holes and fix the barriers, so the whole system keeps working smoothly. (And by the way, fasting physiology also helps the stem cells in your gut regenerate and repair the gut wall, so energy-sucking inflammation there gets dialed down too.)[27]

Now contrast this with what's likely happening in your body right now. Multiple fuels, fats, carbs, and proteins arriving simultaneously and relentlessly, from sunup to sundown and beyond, then taking additional time for digestion, absorption, and processing into ATP, keeping you in the "feeding state" for hours past the optimal cutoff. Remember, the average person is eating food almost continuously for sixteen hours a day, giving your poor overworked mitochondria and gut little time to catch up, much less have any downtime for some R&R.

How to Make Ketones

Your liver produces ketones anytime the supply of glucose is too low for the brain's energetic needs. This can occur during a fasting window of at least twelve hours; when dietary carbohydrates are removed from the diet almost completely (i.e., what's commonly known as a low-carb or keto diet); in the absence of significant amounts of protein; during periods of prolonged, strenuous exercise; or during actual starvation (which I'm hoping you do not experience). If you want to give your body a little nudge into making ketones, you can also consume certain premade ketone supplements and/or fats that can be converted into ketones in your liver. In other words, there are a few ways to "trick" your body into stepping up the ketone-production game, and in the Energy Paradox Program you will use a daily fasting window plus a few bonus strategies to get there!

The Optimal Eating Window

Right about now you're probably wondering just how long your daily feeding and fasting windows need to be to get all these benefits. As a general rule, I recommend you eat your daily meals within a period of no more than twelve hours and, ideally, land on a "sweet spot" of about six to eight hours. That sweet spot could look like having a first meal at 10 a.m. and finishing your last meal (or beverage, apart from water or tea) at 6 p.m., leaving a whopping sixteen hours of fasting in between. Or maybe you're a morning person. You could eat your first meal at 7 a.m. and finish eating at 3 p.m. Woah, that's draconian! But before you throw this book out the window, I beg you for some patience. I'm going to show you lots of options for using chrono consumption to get your energy back. Like Mark Twain said: "Habit is habit and not to be flung out of the window, but coaxed downstairs, one step at time."

So, still with me? Okay, listen, I'm not going to have you starting out eating only six hours a day. That sort of jump would be too challenging for probably 80 percent of you who, like many of my patients when I first meet them, have struggled to make such a giant leap. It's a phenomenon I see regularly when people launch into keto or intermittent fasting diets from a standing stop. They are insulin resistant and don't yet have the metabolic flexibility to start accessing free fatty acids the moment glucose runs out, and thus have a few days of total loss of energy, headaches, and impaired exercise performance as fuel sources fail them. For many people, this discomfort sabotages their efforts and they give up before they've gained any benefit! Rest assured, that's not going to happen with this plan. In Part II, we are going to step down to step up, one hour at a time, until we get to your goals. Now, here's the really good news: You don't have to change your caloric intake; you are not going on a "diet." Instead, I'd like you to think about taking your mitochondria for a six-week spa treatment. And, if you're already eating a relatively healthful diet free of hazardous industrial fats and sugars, or have tried keto, or vegan, or carnivore without much success, and are still feeling sluggish, weighed down, or cloudy, you will come to see how mastering the art of meal timing will finally get you the results you've been looking for.

The Keto Paradox

Okay, I'm sure some of you eager beavers who have tried keto diets are dying to ask me: If making ketones for fuel is so good for me, shouldn't I do it 24/7, 365 days a year by rigorously following a very low-carbohydrate diet and staying in ketosis? (That's the physiological state in which you are always producing a significant number of ketones, not just cycling in and out of making them on a feed-fast rhythm as I described.) My answer: No way.

It's time to challenge the party line that long-term ketogenic diets are good for you because they let you "burn clean energy." And apparently that it is necessary to eat a very low-carb diet because so many of us today (up to 75 percent is frequently cited) are "carbohydrate intolerant." Even my good friend Dr. Mark Hyman has tweeted this statistic. I've seen this repeated so much that I sought out the reference for it, and found it. Lo and behold, it's a misreading of the data. The paper this statistic comes from has nothing to do with carbohydrate intolerance; it's saying 75 percent of people in the world are *lactose* intolerant because they don't have the gene to make lactase, which breaks down the milk sugar lactose.[28] Now, because lactose is a carbohydrate, yes, connect the dots, we get to 75 percent of people are "carbohydrate intolerant." Hey, I was on the Yale Debate Team; I know a hilariously spurious argument when I see one. So, sorry about that, but *none of us are intrinsically carbohydrate intolerant.* And just for a reminder, that's why the Duke rice diet or Okinawan diet of essentially 85 to 100 percent carbohydrates can work, even in diabetics, by selecting one fuel and one fuel only for the mitochondrial assembly line to work on at a time.

Now, don't get me wrong, I am not anti-keto, any more than I am pro the Duke rice diet. Let's just say that the standard ketogenic diet (in other words, a high-fat, low-carb, *low-fiber* diet done *without time-restricted feeding*) doesn't look very good in terms of promoting mitochondrial health or gaining or even preserving long-term muscle mass, and doesn't tend to give you more energy; which may explain why so many people eventually give up on the keto diet. In fact, a long-term high-fat ketogenic diet leads to inflammation, weight gain, and insulin resistance, the very thing most people adopt a ketogenic diet to treat or avoid![29,30,31] Further, the tunnel vision on macronutrients like fat makes many forget to feed their gut buddies the sufficient diversity of fiber they need to make postbiotics for you.

So, unlike what you have been led to believe, following a ketogenic diet has nothing to do with burning fuel-efficient ketones; it has to do with the signaling function of the ketones BHB and acetyl-CoA telling your mitochondria that food is scarce right now, so, guess what, it's time to make more of you guys because hard times are here. Sadly, we've missed what ketones and butyrate are actually telling the mitochondria! The mitochondria are not becoming more efficient because they are *burning* the ketones; they're becoming less efficient while simultaneously adding more of them (workers) to the assembly line, to stop injuring themselves, because otherwise the organism is going to die. (You can prove this by just giving normally fed animals or humans ketones as a pill or drink, and they will have all these effects on mitochondria as if they were actually fasting.)[32]

Remember, in nature, chronic ketosis would only occur during starvation, with its resultant suppression of protein synthesis and accompanying muscle wasting, because you can't even make enough ketones to keep your brain happy, so you borrow proteins from your muscles to manufacture glucose in your liver via *gluconeogenesis*. Which means when you force yourself to stay in ketosis 24/7, 365 days a year, you are at risk of getting overly lean or even wasted.[33] Ketosis follows the same hormetic curve we've discussed where none is bad, a little is just right, and a lot is, quite frankly, horrible. In C², you are going to be in that "sweet spot" where ketones circulate as signaling molecules telling your cells to do necessary repair work and to maximize your mitochondria's safety and health. You'll follow the naturally fluctuating rhythms your body expects: During the controlled eating period, your glucose levels will increase, ketone levels will lower, and cells will increase protein synthesis, undergoing growth and repair—so that you don't experience muscle mass loss or wasting. You don't stay in the state where messages say "famine is nigh!"—these signals fade out before returning the next day. Which means your clocks will be synced, and your metabolism will swing back and forth between the two equally necessary parts of the equation, with utmost flexibility, ergo, optimal energy production. Feed for a few hours, don't eat for a few more hours, before starting it all again. And, as a bonus, take the weekends off. Simple!

Move It to Boost It

There's one more nuance to chrono consumption that I want to stress: Exercise can boost all of the benefits of fasting, helping you train your metabolism to be fit and flexible, and creating conditions where your cellular and mitochondrial cleanup run at their peak. You see, exercise is another challenge that forces your cells to adapt and get resilient—it is another form of hormesis your DNA has evolved to expect. I know that some of you may feel too tired to even want to get moving—I can practically hear your resistance!—but trust me, movement matters.

Your muscles are your metabolic organs, and the main customers for sugars and fats, ready to work for your energy production system if you use them. Think of them as your fuel reserve tanks that eat up glucose swiftly after you consume food, then store extra for you in the form of glycogen. Eighty percent of the glucose you eat actually gets deposited there for safekeeping until you need it. Exercise requires tapping those glucose stores, pushing your body to use them up faster, thereby depleting stored glycogen and getting to the "switching point" where you burn free fatty acids much faster. And the right kind of exercise builds more muscle mass, creating more storage tanks. Meanwhile, it also stimulates muscles to secrete myokines—messenger chemicals that not only regulate hormones that improve insulin sensitivity but stimulate neuronal health in the brain. Furthermore, exercise improves insulin sensitivity by having muscles burn through their glycogen stores and then have to use free fatty acids for fuel, thus increasing your metabolic flexibility (exactly what you want to do to have more energy). The more vigorous the exercise is, the more this effect compounds.

Now imagine following a timed eating protocol where you start the day in a prolonged fasted state, and add some exercise into the mix. It all gets better: First, using your muscles in a fasted state promotes greater mitogenesis and hence greater energy production. (Remember the Stanford study in which only the *non*-insulin-resistant exercisers saw benefits?) The jury is still out on exactly what kinds of exercise promote how much mitochondrial replication,[34] but when you're just starting out, any kind of exercise will offer benefits. Strength training or resistance training seems a very effective way to promote mitogenesis, and I recommend everybody include it in their fitness regimen a few times a week, whether via bodyweight exercises or weight training.

However—and this is a key caveat—consuming food prior to exercise will block most or all of these benefits![35] Now, the fitter and stronger you are, the less you will achieve mitogenesis in your workouts, because you have already met lots of challenges and made large adaptations. That's where working out in the fasted state comes in (i.e., ideally after fasting all night and before your first meal of the day). For already fit folks with some muscle power established, fasting plus exercise works synergistically to increase metabolic flexibility and mitogenesis further, truly giving you the bang for the buck. (Don't slurp a recovery shake the minute you set down that barbell either. You want to give your body some time in the post-workout fasted state to really reap the gains, so please wait at least twenty minutes before eating!)

Second, during exercise your brain increases production of proteins called *neurotrophic factors* (often written as BDNF and FGF), both of which promote the growth of dendrites and axons, boost the formation and strengthening of synapses, and even help to generate new neurons. Guess what this translates to? A better mood and clearer thinking! Paradoxically—and wonderfully so—you are using up energy, and feeling more energized in return.[36]

The other "M" in the M^2 part of our $E = M^2C^2$ energy equation also plays a role here. Have you ever wondered why some people exercise daily and look lean while others doing the same routines don't seem to get the same benefits? It turns out that your gut buddies determine whether your body will respond favorably to exercise or not. In fact, in patients with type 2 diabetes, the effect of exercise sadly is dependent on their microbiome composition.[37] Those with a healthy and diverse microbiome become sensitive to insulin and lose weight when they adopt an exercise program; but those with microbial imbalances see fewer benefits. So, yes, it is all connected. You need exercise to master the energy equation, and you need a healthy gut microbiome to reap the most benefits from exercise. If you've ever stuck with an exercise program but been frustrated by poor results, I hope this gives you hope. Maybe it wasn't you, it was your gut buddies! Don't worry, this program will get them in shape too.

Got Meat? Get Moving!

I know we've been talking about energy, but I can't resist sharing another reason why the effect of exercise on your microbiome matters so much—especially if you eat significant amounts of meat. Our cells coordinate much of their work of growth, metabolism, and maintenance through sensors called *mTOR*. When this signaling pathway gets dysregulated, you age more rapidly and are more susceptible to disease. Those of us who study longevity have long known that diets overly high in animal protein overstimulate mTOR (much more so than plant protein) and mess up its messaging, which is why if you want to live long, you should lay off excessive animal protein. Yet we also now know that exercise boosts certain gut bugs that break down the branch chain amino acids (building blocks of meat protein) that cause this overstimulation.[38] In other words, exercise *protects* you from the potential downsides of too much meat consumption. This explains why many who follow a "primal" or paleo diet, profuse with grass-finished meat, subvert longevity experts' expectations and boast vital good health: These folks typically lift heavy weights, sprint hard, and maintain enviable workout routines. (Though we don't yet know how long they'll live! The paleo movement is still quite new.) All this to say, your gut buddies have you covered, if you give them the active lifestyle that they need.

So there you have it. You've learned about all the ways we have ended up overfed, underpowered, and in something of a funk, to boot. You've learned that to get your energy back online and revving as it should, there are two Ms to take care of—your microbiome and your mitochondria—and a pair of Cs to master in a new kind of eating pattern called chrono consumption. Together that gets you to E: Energy! Over the course of the next few weeks, you can start to establish new habits that will end your chronic energy slump, put the pep back in your step, and set you on a better course that you can maintain for a lifetime. Ready to get started? Let's seize the day. It's time for your get-up-and-go to get back for good.

ENERGY MYTH #6: The Menopausal/ Manopausal Myth

My institutes are located in two hotbeds of antiaging medicine: Palm Springs and Santa Barbara, California. And without exaggeration I can attest that hormone clinics seem as ubiquitous in Southern California as coffee shops are in Seattle or Portland. Why? There is a pervasive myth that with a certain stage in life comes a "natural" decline in energy, along with mental sharpness, and perhaps lust (for life and other things) as well. We've become mistakenly fixated on the idea that regaining the sex hormone levels of a twenty-five-year-old—estrogen, progesterone, and testosterone for women; testosterone and growth hormones for men—is the key to energy, sex drive, and endurance. I understand; the siren song of youth is hard to resist. But it's misguided, and sadly, I have had a first-row view of the havoc hormone replacement can wreak in both women and men, from "man boobs" in men to women literally shaving their arms and faces. And it can also promote the development of hormone-sensitive cancers such as breast, ovarian, and prostate cancer, as I have seen in many patients who are newly arrived at my clinics seeking treatment for their cancer while taking these hormones. (In addition, the jury is still out whether testosterone replacement is actually effective in improving performance, energy, or muscle mass in elderly men.)[39]

I am not anti–hormone therapy, and in fact I prescribe it when justified by bloodwork and/or symptoms. But it is certainly not my go-to solution for flagging energy levels. In my practice I see about 5 percent of postmenopausal women who are profoundly sensitive to the lack of estrogen; the unrelenting hot flashes, the brain dysfunction that clears with tiny (and I do mean tiny) doses of topical estrogen. And yes, about 15 percent of women will respond to tiny bits of testosterone with an improved sex drive, but if it doesn't kick in at a low dose, enough testosterone to grow a beard isn't the answer to a poor love life. And often the lack of sex drive may be driven by the lack of energy we are addressing in this book. And here's a shocker: I have never met a man with low "T" who doesn't have insulin resistance and an elevated insulin level. Ever. And, I have never had to give a man testosterone to boost his levels; I just had to teach him how to eat and those low levels improved back to normal.

Finally, I like to remind my patients looking for the antiaging cure that none of the centenarians in the Blue Zones were ever on hormone replacement; they seem to have done just fine (and may I suggest, perhaps even better?) without it. In conclusion, there are better ways to get your energy back, and that's why you are here!

The 7 Deadly (Energy) Disruptors

I can't let you leap into the Energy Paradox Program until you've taken a quick tour of the most challenging *external* forces exerting pressure on your energy levels and overall health. If you're familiar with the *Paradox* books, you probably have a pretty good understanding of the role these bad guys play in setting you up for a host of illnesses. For those of you who are new to this idea, let me offer a brief summary of how these insidious offenders make you sick and set you up for an energy crisis.

The external Energy Disruptors range from industrial chemicals to unsuitable foods to toxic environmental influences. These seemingly mundane things we encounter every day can create an invisible storm of hormonal confusion and intestinal and microbiome damage. Collectively, they add up to quite a shock to your normal operating system. Some of them weaken and injure the gut wall, making it permeable; some can cause radical imbalances in the gut ecosystem, wiping out valuable gut buddies and generating gut inflammation; and still others create conditions where the natural ingredients our body requires to produce energy suddenly go missing, or worse, exert invisible stress and damage on your mitochondria.

Overwhelming as it may seem to tackle disruptors you unknowingly eat, breathe in, or live among daily, I promise there are ways to downgrade them to mere annoyances that no longer derail your energy (I'll share the strategies for avoiding or reducing their impact in Part II). Once you know better, you can do better.

Energy Disruptor #1: Antibiotics

I'm detailing throughout this book the advantages of a *pro-*, *pre-*, and *post*biotic diet and lifestyle. But here's the inconvenient truth: We are awash in *anti*biotics today. Both in our medical system, where eight million pounds of antibiotics are prescribed to Americans annually, and—less obviously—in our food system, where almost five times that amount is given to animals in the effort to fatten them quicker for slaughter.

Broad-spectrum antibiotics—the type we are most often exposed to—work by killing almost all strains of bacteria simultaneously. Capable of countering life-threatening infections, they were a miracle when introduced almost sixty years ago. Yet these bacteria blasters have become a vastly overused crutch, used in milder situations where their firepower is not warranted. (The most rampant misuse is when doctors prescribe antibiotics for *viral* infections, like that cough or runny nose.) This crutch is now showing its unintended consequences: We know that early antibiotic use in children (even in utero exposure) is associated with obesity later in life, as well as behavioral challenges, allergies, autoimmunity, and other diseases.[40,41] The same effects play out in adults, with many conditions such as diabetes, IBD, autoimmune diseases, depression—and, not surprisingly, unshakable fatigue—linked to antibiotic overuse.

Taking a broad-spectrum antibiotic is the human equivalent of burning down the entire rain forest to tame one invasive species. Without the ecosystem working as a whole, the normal development of immune cells is stunted, nutritional deficiencies can arise, and, most important, the bacterial diversity in the gut microbiome is wiped out. The net effect is also impaired immunity that makes you more vulnerable to pathogens. In addition, the bacteria that do survive develop antibiotic resistance and, to make matters worse, antibiotics can also impact your mitochondria, which, after all, are really bacteria too. Bacteria meet antibiotic: Not a marriage made in heaven. Studies now show that commonly prescribed antibiotics can directly hurt your energy systems. They can drive mitochondrial dysfunction and damage by promoting high oxidative stress.[42] They have even been shown to have a dramatic effect on mitochondrial DNA, causing potentially severe health problems— that I've witnessed in my own patients.[43] Certain classes of antibiotics have also been shown to damage neurons, creating behavioral and neurological issues such as depression and anxiety.[44,45] (By the way, it's been shown that antibiotics wipe out most of the neuroprotective benefits of intermittent fasting[46]—a cornerstone of the program you'll be following in the Energy Paradox Program!) And I can virtually guarantee you that your well-meaning health care provider knows little about these side effects.

Unfortunately, you are exposed to antibiotics every day even without taking them in pill form. The vast majority of antibiotics in the US actually go into animal feed, either used prophylactically to shield the animals against disease or to fatten them for slaughter quickly. This should be one of your major motivations to seek out antibiotic-free animal protein (organic certification guarantees this; other nonorganic products may be labeled antibiotic-free). Unfortunately, we also know that antibiotic residues leach out of the feedlot and into crops[47] (sorry, vegetarians).

Obviously, there are times when you need to take prescription antibiotics—just remember, it should be a last resort. Studies now show it can take up to two years for your body to regain most of the energy-supporting ecosystem that you lose after a course of antibiotics—and some strains of microbes never recover at all.[48]

Energy Disruptor #2: Glyphosate (Roundup)

You may already be concerned about the world's most widely used herbicide, Roundup, and its chemical cousins. And rightly so. Its active ingredient glyphosate, coupled with other formulants that make it cling to leaves, is, I believe, one of the most dangerous but ubiquitous chemicals in our food and water system today. After studying it for years, I'm becoming increasingly convinced it may be the worst disruptor of all when it comes to our energy systems and health at large. Glyphosate is essentially an antibiotic against the earth. It kills plants by disrupting a metabolic pathway called the *shikimate pathway*, which is present in all bacteria, fungi, and plants, that synthesizes amino acids into proteins, the building blocks of life.[49,50] It was formulated for use on crops that have been designed to resist its action (these are genetically modified organisms, or GMO crops), ensuring by a canny twist that only the surrounding nonengineered plants, aka natural weeds, would die. However, it is now a widespread conventional farming practice to use Roundup as a desiccant on non-GMO crops like most corn, wheat, oats, and canola. This means that glyphosate is sprayed on these crops just prior to harvest so that the stalks are dry and more efficient to harvest and process. So, those of you looking for the non-GMO label, look again. Your "safe" grains are covered in toxic chemicals.

Roundup was long touted as nontoxic to animals and humans, on the basis that its lethal pathway only attacks plants. That's the first red flag: As you know by now, *you* are home to thousands of strains of bacteria that are pivotal to your survival and energy— and guess what, they all use the shikimate pathway! This product easily destroys them just like a weed.

A twenty-three-year-long study in California tracked glyphosate levels in urine and found that our bodies are showing dramatic increases in the chemical.[51] This directly impacts your energy levels (and obviously your health as a whole) for myriad reasons. Glyphosate appears to make the tight junctions of the intestinal wall more permeable, as well as the tight junctions holding the blood-brain barrier together.[52] Imagine the total effect: Gut flora are assaulted, leaky gut and inflammation are rampant, and the blood-brain barrier starts to leak inflammatory compounds into the brain as well—no wonder your energy tanks and your cognition gets weaker. (Worryingly, many connect the epidemic levels of neuroinflammatory and neurodegenerative diseases to our ever-increasing glyphosate burden.) Equally nefariously, glyphosate strips micronutrients out of the foods you eat, leaving your body deficient in critical cofactors for energy. It also suppresses an enzyme that you need to have adequate vitamin D in your body (remember, that helps heal your gut), and in synergy with other ingredients in herbicides, it is a mitochondrial toxin, causing a collapse of transmembrane electrical potential in animal studies as well as mitochondrial swelling.[53]

I hate to say it, because I'm an optimist, but it's everywhere today, even if you already try to avoid GMO grains and legumes. A few reasons why: Most of the animal products you buy, unless stated otherwise (i.e., labeled organic or certifiably 100 percent grass-fed and grass-finished or pasture-raised) have chowed on these chemicals in grain-based feed—which then make their way into you. Plus, the desiccant is not magically "washed off" those grain-based non-GMO products you and your kids might eat, in your cereal, bread, oatmeal, or crackers—and if the outer husks are left on for "whole-grain goodness," you get extra exposure. Last, many products we enjoy, like beer, wine, and honey, contain glyphosate too, so the unknown exposures add up. I wish I could click my fingers and make it go away, but for now, the onus is on you, the consumer, to think carefully about what you buy and how it was produced. The old adage "know your farmer" has never been more important. (As a father and grandfather myself, I'd be remiss not to point out that Roundup has massive application on non-farmland green spaces, like parks, school grounds, golf courses, heck, your own backyard or sidewalk. For more information on the recreational areas near you, follow the work of nontoxiccommunities.com.)

Energy Disruptor #3: Environmental Chemicals

Glyphosate isn't the only chemical we need to worry about; exposure to hundreds of chemicals of manmade origin is unavoidable today. More than one hundred thousand new chemicals have been introduced into our environment in the form of industrial and consumer products over recent decades.[54] They pervade our homes, workplaces, food supply, and even our air, soil, and water, and at least three hundred of them or their metabolites have been measured in human biological samples. You're likely familiar with many of the categories of concerns—plastic-industry chemicals like bisphenols and phthalates, persistent organic pollutants and heavy metals, and, of course, pesticides, herbicides, and biocides, not to mention the fact that microplastics are even found in the plants we eat, which increase heavy metal loads in us.[55] Though many are known as endocrine disruptors—they throw off the delicate balance of thyroid, insulin, and reproductive hormones and more—and are associated with poor health outcomes, only fairly recently have scientists parsed how many of these effects may be mediated by the microbiome. It's beyond the scope of this book to break down every category of hazardous environmental chemical in detail. But it is crucial to take a broad-strokes look at how much these chemicals impair your energy potential.

First, most of these environmental chemicals appear to alter the gut microbiota. We know that exposure to chemicals like the plasticizer bisphenol A (BPA), which can leach out of food cans, microwaveable packaging, and some plastic bottles, reduces the gut buddies that make short-chain fatty acids and creates chronic intestinal and liver inflammation and metabolic disorder. BPA and its partner in crime, phthalates, also block receptors for thyroid hormone, even at low doses. Unfortunately, alternatives used (so that a product can be labeled "BPA-free") are typically even less studied, rendering them potentially worse. Meanwhile, exposure to some of the industrial chemicals used in agriculture, in fast food packaging, and nonstick coatings for cookware have been shown to change the composition of the microbiome and incite inflammation in the intestines. Given how many Americans eat nonorganic food, fast food, and fried food, is it any wonder everyone's so tuckered out?

Second, many endocrine-disrupting chemical offenders you encounter daily are proved to be inflammatory.[56] This may be partly because of the biome changes. As you know by now, inflammation drives not only obesity and immune dysregulation but also plain old fatigue.

In my deadly disruptor hall of fame, I have a special place for food preservatives, some of which stimulate the immune system; one in particular is TBHQ, a preservative used in most commercial seed oils and a lot of packaged fried foods.

Another hall of famer is chemical-based sunscreen. Research has shown that UV-filtering chemicals like oxybenzone absorb directly from your skin into your blood after one application, and by mimicking the effect of your natural hormones, disturb the vital and delicate hormone balance in your body.[57] I've shared how chemical sunscreens lower your ability to convert vitamin D into its active form; we're also learning that direct sunlight exposure on skin has a positive effect on the intestinal microbiome, suggesting there is a skin-gut axis at work that helps support the health of your microbiome.[58] Your gut, it turns out, needs sunlight to thrive—just please monitor your exposure.

Environmental chemicals even alter your thyroid function.[59] Sadly, your thyroid gland is exquisitely sensitive to the action of endocrine disruptors. It is also extraordinarily important for your functioning, cognitive clarity, and all-around get-up-and-go!

You can find out more about the most common environmental chemicals online (the Environmental Working Group's website is a great place to start). And for a full list of products to avoid and safer alternatives, see *The Plant Paradox.*

Energy Disruptor #4: Overused Pharmaceutical Drugs

I am not against the use of pharmaceutical drugs, prescription or over-the-counter versions. They are sometimes essential, and other times can be a bridge to get you to a place where you no longer need their help. But relying on them long-term rather than resolving the root cause of the issue they are treating can throw a wrench into your energy systems. Given that our tired nation fills 4.38 billion (yes, billion) prescriptions per year and buys an additional 32.2 billion dollars' worth of over-the-counter meds[60] (most of which used to be prescription only), if you want to solve the Energy Paradox, it's important to look at the pills you pop.

Along with antibiotics, some of the worst energy offenders include the vastly overused nonsteroidal anti-inflammatory drugs (NSAIDs) like ibuprofen (such as Advil and Motrin), naproxen (used in Aleve), Celebrex, Voltaren, and others. I call them "hand grenades" for your gut; they damage the mucosal barrier in the small intestine and colon, allowing lectins, LPSs, and other foreign substances to pass through the intestinal wall and initiate the inflammatory cascade—which, ironically, will make you reach for more of them to dull the hurt.

The second problematic group is proton pump inhibitors (PPIs) or other acid-blocking drugs, like Prilosec, Nexium, Protonix, and Zantac. Often used to relieve discomfort after eating, these drugs reduce levels of stomach acid, and in so doing, strip you of an important acid buffer against lectins and less-helpful microbes seeking to gain more real estate. Guess what happens when they're not kept in check? Leaky gut and inflammation, and sometimes uncomfortable symptoms due to small intestinal bacterial overgrowth (SIBO). They can also foster incomplete protein digestion, which in turn allows more protein-containing lectins into your intestine as well as prevents you from absorbing proteins that you do need in your small bowel. But here's the worst news: These drugs not only affect the proton pumps in your stomach cells that produce acid, they affect the proton pumps inside all your cells and in your mitochondria, invisibly but palpably slowing down energy production; they also have a special ability to cross the blood-brain barrier and poison your brain's mitochondria, contributing to brain fog, cognitive slowdown, and dementia.[61]

PPIs aren't the only drugs that hit your mitochondria hard. Many side effects of pharmaceutical medications are now linked to mito-chondrial impairment[62]—affecting older patients in particular. Mitochondrial-linked organ toxicities are the most common rea-son for prescription medications to be given black box warnings. In addition to the previously mentioned antibiotics, antidepressants like selective serotonin reuptake inhibitors (SSRIs) receive these warnings. They act to increase the concentration of serotonin by blocking reabsorption, but meanwhile exert unintended effects on mitochondria. Some research has shown that antidepressants also reduce the number and diversity of gut bacteria.[63]

Another area of medication overuse is hormonal birth control pills. I am in no position to tell any woman how to manage her reproductive health, but I do think it's important to give women who may be considering taking this medication all of the facts, as physicians fail to do so when prescribing "the pill." Studies show that up to 50 percent of birth control medication escapes the small intestine, where it is supposed to be absorbed, and ends up in the large intestine, where it can significantly diminish the micro-biome. The effect may even be akin to that of antibiotics—and think how many years a woman can be on the pill! Furthermore, this medication depletes antioxidants, including a compound found in all your cells and tissues called CoQ10, that are crucial to mitochondrial energy production and that naturally decline with age—making CoQ10 supplementation important if you are on the pill. (Vitamin C, vitamin B_6, folate, B_{12}, zinc, and magnesium should also be supported.)

The depletion of CoQ10 is not only relegated to hormonal birth control. The very commonly prescribed statin drugs block the production of this mitochondrial driver (along with several other essential nutrients). Statins interfere with vitamin K_2 and D_3 metabolism, probably because they change the microbiome, and there is increasing evidence that statin drugs increase the risk of diabetes. While I do prescribe these drugs in serious cases, I like to help the patient transform their diet, restore proper mitochondrial function, and arrive at a place where they do not need them, because if you don't need them, why take them?

Another category of offenders is prescribed sleep aids. It's no surprise that by some estimates up to seventy million Americans use sleep medication and/or have insomnia. But the truth is that these medications are a horrible disruptor in their own right. News flash: Sleep drugs don't allow for normal sleep. They're technically in the category of *sedative hypnotics*, and they work by artificially stimulating production of the calming neurotransmitter GABA—essentially knocking out your cortex (your thinking brain). This is exceedingly different from the intricate choreography of natural sleep in which many different brain phases occur and, alarmingly, the consequence of use is a very real increased risk of dementia.[64]

The good news for those sleepless nights is that chronic inflammation interferes with sleep, so when you remedy the inflammation, you will win significant improvements in your sleep.

Energy Disruptor #5: Fructose

I say this phrase so often, I should really make a T-shirt with it: *Give Fructose the Boot.* Fructose is the sugar that naturally occurs in fruits, honey, maple syrup, sugar cane, sugar beets, and corn, and even vegetables that have seeds, which are technically fruits. Our diets are loaded with fructose, and I don't mean only from processed foods and drinks containing high-fructose corn syrup. Fruit smoothies and juices are also sources of fructose in our diets. Sadly, today, our fruit is bigger, and higher in fructose than ever—it's been engineered to be sweeter and give consumers more incentive to buy.

I've long been fanatical about how dangerous fructose is in promoting aging and how it tricks your body into believing it's summer all year, thereby cueing it to "pack on the pounds for winter." But fructose's effect on you, your liver, and your mitochondria deserves a closer look. Fructose, unlike glucose, is absorbed from your intestines and taken, for the most part, directly to your liver. There, it prevents adenosine monophosphate (AMP) from entering the ATP production chain in your mitochondria. Instead, AMP gets shuttled into the production of uric acid, the cause of gout, some kidney stones, and high blood pressure. But that's not its worst effect. In your liver, it is turned into the saturated fatty acid palmitate.[65] As you read in Chapter 4, palmitate is what your cells use to produce ceramides, the waxy lipid that keeps your fat cells from exploding but causes insulin resistance in an effort to protect your poor mitochondria from overworking. If that wasn't enough, fructose is a major contributor to the epidemic of nonalcoholic fatty liver disease (NAFLD) or nonalcoholic steatohepatitis (NASH). Palmitate is incorporated into triglycerides, which promote the production of small dense LDLs and the suppression of HDL production, not exactly what you'd hope for from that glass of orange juice. To recap: Fructose is bad, it's a direct mitochondrial toxin,[66] and a major driver of heart disease. Indeed, I found that removal of "healthy" fruits from the diet dramatically lowered risk factors for heart disease in a paper I presented to the American Heart Association in 2008. Shocking as it may sound, that fruit smoothie and processed protein bar in the morning is actually making *you produce less energy*, contributing to more inflammation, as well as doing a number on your liver and heart.

Energy Disruptor #6: Junk Light

First there was junk food to worry about. Now there's junk light. We're learning more about it via the science of photobiology, which studies the influence of light on biological organisms. One of its surprising findings is that the light bulb may be one of the biggest health hazards ever invented (sorry, Mr. Edison). The hazards come partly because artificial light has "artificially" allowed us to manipulate our light exposure. This disrupts the fundamental relationship between all life-forms and the sun; light is the fundamental driver of your circadian rhythm, which regulates all of your metabolic functions.

We humans are very subtly attuned to the full spectrum of sunlight. Not simply the shift from darkness to light—as was once thought—but actually to the shifts in color spectrum as fire-like early morning light turns bluer, and then later in the day, as blue turns red again at sunset. The relative increase and decrease of blue content in daylight is an important signal to the circadian clock system in your body, which cues all kinds of energy-making or energy-conserving activities. (We will discuss this in greater detail in Chapter 8; when you finish this book you will be a certified circadian rhythm master!)

Light biologist Dr. Alexander Wunsch has described how the shortest wavelengths in natural light—the blue colors you see in full daylight along with invisible ultraviolet light—induce high stress at the cellular level.[67] Wunsch found that as the amount of blue increases, you produce "remedies" for the potential downside of excessive UV exposure—such as cortisol to reduce inflammation from burning and vasoactive substances like adrenaline to counter any burn. That's right—blue light causes the body to produce stress hormones! Now, eons ago, if you were roaming naked outside while this happened, those hormones would have helped to protect us. But when sitting fully clothed under fluorescent lights in your office, the effects are not so great. This light-induced stress piles on to the already high levels of stress from our sedentary, indoor lifestyles and compounds the inflammation and exhaustion it can cause.

Now imagine you keep the lights on 24/7 (or somewhere in that ballpark) and add in the blue light from computer screens and devices. You've not only been overexposed to the blue and invisible UV wavelengths, you've now cut out the red wavelengths of nature. This matters because the red wavelengths (infrared and near-infrared light) are shown to help to *boost* mitochondria.[68] Without it, you're overexposed to only one fraction of the full spectrum of light your ancient biology expects. And all that blue light after sunset also disrupts the key signaling molecule melatonin, which signals your nervous system (via your circadian clock) to switch into rest and repair mode. It can push back melatonin's normal production—key for sleep onset—by more than three hours. And, without sleep, the body's regenerative programs are much harder to run. Melatonin also balances out all that immune-suppressing and blood-sugar-elevating cortisol you may have generated earlier—you really want it! Light received through the eyes also helps the production of the motivation hormone *dopamine*. Light biologists point out another fatiguing effect of modern light sources: Many emit invisible "flickers," which also create a stress response as your brain works hard to adapt to the inconsistency and make it seem consistent. Tired, struggling with sleep, and low in mojo? That all-day, all-night glow may be partly to blame.

Basically, we are overlit, overstimulated, and overstressed. You can't escape it entirely, but just like you can choose healthier options to junk food, you can say no to junk light as much as you can.

Energy Disruptor #7: Electromagnetic Fields (EMFs)

We are living in an unseen soup of electro smog. The frequencies that come from the wireless communications systems we depend upon for connection are stressors our ancestors could not have imagined. Sure, those guys were bathed in the naturally occurring electromagnetic wavelengths of light from the sun. But today's manmade (or "nonnative") electromagnetic frequencies that transmit data to our devices and between cell towers with pulsing, lower amplitude signals are quite different in their signature. Some people are canaries in the coalmine, including several of my own patients: Those who are especially sensitive to EMFs experience fatigue, brain fog, and headaches when around unchecked levels of these frequencies—say in an apartment building riddled with routers, smart meters, or a cell tower nearby. (Estimates are that about 20 percent of people may be sensitive in this way.) But the rest of us are still affected, and mainly unaware of the effects happening at the cellular level.

The radio frequencies that carry data around our communications systems occupy the microwave part of the electromagnetic spectrum. This means they are capable of causing heat production in tissues. Yet research is showing many other nonthermal biological effects that, until now, have escaped regulation by the telecommunication governing board, the FTC. These cause a level of interference to normal signaling in the body that hurts your mitochondria and may be a factor in your tiredness, cognitive fuzz, and nighttime tossing and turning.[69]

According to Martin Pall, professor emeritus of biochemistry at Washington State University, electromagnetic radiation of all kinds (including the extremely low frequency fields thrown off by electricity lines) wreak cellular havoc by changing the voltage gate that regulates how much calcium can get into the cell. Simply stated, too much calcium is problematic, but so is too little. Electromagnetic fields overactivate these gates and flood the cells with calcium. This injury catalyzes a dramatic cellular survival response: A little-known free radical called *peroxynitrite* is released that spikes significant oxidative damage, hurting the delicate membranes of the cells and mitochondria and their DNA and damaging gene expression.[70]

Okay, so far, so bad. But it could get worse. The looming new fifth generation telecommunications network (5G) is poised to introduce a new layer of millimeter wave signaling that cycles at infinitely faster speeds on top of the existing frequencies, so that more data transfer can occur, faster than ever. (Note: This is not the same thing as 5.6 Ghz on your router.) Information on this technology is sparse—it is perhaps purposefully shrouded in mystery. Even the prestigious *Scientific American* recently opined that the health risks of this unstudied technology warranted pause on its rollout. As I write this, several cities, including Santa Barbara, where one of my offices is located, have put a hold on 5G.

The good news is that you can mitigate a great deal of this effect by changing the way you use your devices at home and work and setting up your workstation properly. I also advocate something few people know about: outwitting the calcium flux mischief maker by taking potassium magnesium supplements daily, ideally a mix of oral and topical, as well as consuming sesame oil daily. More on this in Chapter 10.

PART II

THE
ENERGY PARADOX
PROGRAM

CHAPTER 7

THE ENERGY PARADOX
EATING PROGRAM

Now that you know *why* your get-up-and-go got up and gone, it's time to focus on solutions to help you recharge your battery and start feeling like yourself again. That all starts with the foods you eat—and just as important, if not more, the foods you *don't* eat. By eating foods that feed your microbiome—and consequently your mitochondria—and avoiding those that cause damage, we'll reduce inflammation, heal your gut, and rev up ATP production. And that's not all—in this program, we're also going to change up *when* you eat. By following a chrono consumption schedule, you'll give your body the overhaul it needs to improve metabolic flexibility and enhance insulin sensitivity.

The Energy Paradox Program is based on three main objectives: heal your roots; regenerate your soil; and end mitochondrial gridlock. And you know what? It doesn't take that long to improve your gut biome and ATP production, which means that you will notice improvements quickly and be motivated to stay on track.

While you will likely be changing your diet quite a bit (after all, if you were eating and avoiding the right foods, you wouldn't be in an energy crisis!), here's the good news: I'm not going to make you eat anything you don't want to eat. This program is built on flexibility and options, whether you're a vegetarian or a carnivore, a paleo devotee or a vegan. Whatever "camp" or "tribe" you consider yourself to be a part of, you will just expand your horizons as you eat to support your gut buddies. By giving them the things they like—lots of green stuff, some prebiotic fiber from yams, jicama, or artichokes (just a few examples)—and clearing out the things that harm them, such as sugars and bad fats, you will restore proper balance to your microbiome.

Our regimen will also harness the power of ketones. Remember, the signaling power of ketones gets your mitochondria's attention, and in doing so, they react by multiplying to protect you and themselves from perceived stress. But this program is not a keto diet—far from it. Here is where the Goldilocks rule comes into play: You want just the right amount of ketones for the best results. Not making any ketones in a twenty-four-hour day cycle is bad, but remaining in a state of ketosis all the time, day in and day out, is even worse. Keto spoiler alert! If you're in a state of ketosis all the time, you can actually become more inflamed and more insulin resistant.[1] It also causes that dreaded mitochondrial uncoupling, which actually decreases ATP production.[2] That's why the timed eating element of this program will allow your body to hit the "sweet spot" of making enough ketones to promote metabolic flexibility, not prevent it, all the while feeding your bugs the good stuff they need.

What's on the Menu?

So: What does all of this look like on your plate? It starts with eating foods as close to their natural form as possible. The bulk of your diet will be made up of vegetables that contain prebiotic fiber, some nuts and seeds, pressure-cooked lentils and legumes, wild fish, shellfish, and omega-3 eggs. If you desire, you can also enjoy a little grass-fed and grass-finished meat and pastured poultry, and some occasional prebiotic, in-season, low-fructose fruit. (It is also possible—and even encouraged!—to follow this program without eating animal-sourced foods.) Heck, I'll even throw in a glass of red wine or champagne at dinner, and dark chocolate for dessert! I promise you everything here will be delicious, just a bit different from what you currently eat.

Energy Paradox Program Food Rules

This program may look and feel familiar to you if you're a long-time reader of my books. Remember, we're building on the same guiding philosophy of the other Paradox eating regimens (yes, you will still aim to avoid gut-busting lectins at all costs!) and adding foods that will help banish the energy blues and promote energy production. The rules that follow will help you fortify the energy-boosting trifecta of repairing the gut wall, restoring a diverse and thriving microbiome, and restoring insulin sensitivity and metabolic flexibility. I've combined these tenets into five "Dos" and four "Don'ts" to help guide your choices at every meal:

The Dos
Rule 1: Eat Foods Rich in Prebiotic Fiber
Many of you probably take a probiotic supplement to help support the health of your microbiome—and I am a supporter of probiotics, but what is even better is to feed the good bacteria that have been cowering in the far reaches of your gut without the nutrients they need: prebiotic fibers. Foods rich in prebiotic fiber support the health and reproduction of your gut buddies. And when the good guys are finally getting what they want, they'll signal to your brain

that their needs are met, which means that you will literally feel less hungry. And just like with my meat-and-potato-eating patients, you'll also notice that you'll start to crave the kinds of foods that nourish your gut buddies rather than those that don't—and they'll return the favor by nourishing you and your mitochondria.

Indeed, recent studies have found that water-fasting humans who were given about 100 calories of undigestible prebiotic fiber daily as their only food were able to easily fast for seven to fourteen days without hunger.[3] Think about that for a moment. The bugs were fed, and via production of postbiotics, assured their host organism that everything was fine, so no need to look for any more food. Like I've said for the last twenty years, give your gut buddies what they need and they will take care of you.[4] In addition, you'll see a remarkable difference in your digestion and your energy, mood levels, and overall health.

Foods rich in prebiotic fiber include tubers, rutabagas, parsnips, radishes, roots, the chicory family (such as radicchio and endive), okra, artichokes, pressure-cooked beans and legumes, leeks, asparagus, onions, basil seeds, flaxseeds, and more. In addition, two of my preferred sweeteners are Just Like Sugar, which is essentially pure inulin (the same prebiotic fiber found in the chicory family and other gut-friendly vegetables) and allulose, both of which sweeten without any blood sugar–spiking effects while feeding your gut buddies. Another way to get prebiotics is to take powdered psyllium husk or try my new favorite, soaked basil seeds. Start with 1 teaspoon a day in water and work up to 1 tablespoon a day.

Rule 2: Eat Foods That Promote Postbiotic Production

Cruciferous vegetables like broccoli and cauliflower and other sulfur-containing veggies like the allium family (onions, garlic, leeks, chives, shallots, scallions) get top billing in the quest to create the all-important signaling compounds made in your gut. Cruciferous veggies also contain compounds that gut bacteria convert into a postbiotic called *indole*, which has been shown to help prevent fatty liver disease.[5] Many of these foods also donate sulfur molecules, used to make hydrogen sulfide and other postbiotics. Fun tip: When you chop your cruciferous vegetables before cooking, an enzyme called *myrosinase* is released, which has important anticancer properties. It won't be released if you cook first and chop later.

Rule 3: Make Your Starches More Resistant

Resistant starches are so-named because they are "resistant" to fast digestion; they are processed more slowly in your small intestine, and some of them make it downstream to our large intestine, where your gut buddies are waiting to help with the job. Slowing down digestion helps to reduce the mitochondrial fuel bottleneck. Yams, taro root, sorghum, millet, pressure-cooked rice, and cassava can all become resistant starches when they are cooked, then chilled, and then reheated. And before you turn up your nose at reheating "leftovers," consider that many populations who traditionally include rice as a centerpiece of their diet actually eat it reheated, after cooking a large pot to last the week. Smart, huh? You save time in meal prep and get the benefits of eating resistant starch!

But here's a word of warning and a reminder. The more you keep the plant material in its original form, the more resistant it becomes to digestion by you and the more usable it is to your gut buddies. In other words, a whole baked yam cooled offers a lot more resistant starch than sweet potato flour or pasta. While a cassava flour tortilla is vastly preferable to wheat flour or corn tortillas with their high lectin content, it's still a whopping load of quickly digested sugars for your overworked mitochondria. Many root vegetables, such as beets and carrots, start out containing multiple complex carbs and resistant starches, but if you cook them at all, they'll lose their benefit, so it's best to eat them raw if possible.

Rule 4: Eat Fruit Only When in Season, and in Moderation

Fruit didn't earn its nickname "nature's candy" for nothing—it's full of fructose, one of the biggest troublemakers for your mitochondria and liver. And these days thanks to hybridization, fruit is actually bred for sugar content and size. We now have apples that are the size of grapefruit with names like Honeycrisp. What does that tell you? It's pure sugar. A single apple or a cup of seedless grapes has the fructose load of 6 teaspoons of table sugar, which makes a beeline for your liver, slashing ATP production, while making palmitate and hence ceramides to further choke off your mitochondria!

If you're going to eat berries, believe it or not, the modern blueberry has the highest sugar content of any berry; they too have been bred for sugar. If you can find wild blueberries, and you usually have to get them frozen, they're a better choice. Blackberries, followed by raspberries, followed by strawberries have the least sugar content of the berries. In season, pomegranate and passion fruit seeds are actually the best fruits for our purposes. Just be sure to avoid juice in all forms. Drinking juice is basically "mainlining" fructose. Finally, as I always say, when in doubt, give fruit the boot! I suggest treating fruit like dessert and aiming to eat only local, seasonal (preferably during the summer and early fall), and organic.

Rule 5: Enjoy Mitochondrial Must-Haves: Melatonin and Phospholipids

In Part I, you learned that your mitochondria need two special substances to protect them from excessive oxidative stress and optimize their function. The first is melatonin, and the good news is you can get melatonin from the foods you eat. Melatonin-rich foods include pistachios, mushrooms, dark-colored rice (pressure cooked, please), and, very important, a fat that is a cornerstone of the Paradox eating philosophy: olive oil. In one recent study, consuming a liter of olive oil per week was shown to protect against worsening heart disease and dementia in patients with high ceramide levels.[6] Here is a list of foods that contain melatonin, from highest to lowest (ng/grams).[7] While your gut buddies will make melatonin for you by synthesizing amino acids, this extra boost of food-sourced melatonin is a real boost to your mitochondrial energy system, so be sure to include some of these in your diet on a regular basis.

Pistachios 233,000
Mushrooms 4,300–6,400
Black pepper 1092
Red rice 212
Black rice 182
Mustard seeds 129–189
Olive oil 89–119
Brewed coffee 60–80
Red wine 8–129
Cranberries 25–96
Almonds 39
White basmati rice 38.5
Purslane 19
Tart cherries 13.5
Strawberries 5.5–13
Flaxseeds 12

The second mitochondrial optimizer is phospholipids. As you read earlier, these special fats keep the mitochondrial membranes in tip-top shape so that the assembly line of ATP production can function optimally. These are found in high amounts in shellfish such as mussels, scallops, clams, oysters, shrimp, crab, squid, and lobster. I encourage you to add these foods whenever you can. If you can't find them fresh, you can certainly enjoy them canned or frozen.

The Don'ts

The first five rules will help you fill your plate with the best foods for supporting your energy systems. Doing so will automatically help you eat less of the foods you should absolutely avoid—I'm talking about the highly processed foods that come out of a box, or the takeout from your favorite fast food joint. These foods are not only harmful to overall health, but also dramatically decrease energy production,[8] so let's take a closer look at why you should avoid these foods on the Energy Paradox Program.

Rule #6: Leave the Lectins

Breads, pasta, grains and pseudo grains (like amaranth, quinoa, and buckwheat), white potatoes, brown rice, corn, peppers, tomatoes, beans, lentils, and some seeds. (Note: White rice contains a lower lectin load than brown rice; it must be pressure cooked to bring this to acceptable levels. Pressure-cooked black and red rice, both high in melatonin, are acceptable.)

What do these foods have in common? Well, besides the fact that they're probably in almost all your favorite dishes . . . they're also chock-full of lectins. When high-lectin foods were introduced to our diet about ten thousand years ago in the form of grains and beans, our health dramatically changed for the worse. While many people have still never even heard of them, I believe and have published data that lectins are one of the greatest dangers in the American diet. Here are just a few reasons why:

1. **Lectins cause massive digestive damage.** Lectins are difficult to digest (remember, they are a plant's defense system against being eaten—they are meant to cause you discomfort!) and reduce nutrient absorption, cause inflammation, and eliminate gut buddies.

2. **Lectins poke holes in your intestinal walls and leak into your bloodstream.** Lectins are a leading cause of leaky gut, owing to their ability to break the tight junctions that bind one enterocyte to another in that tennis court–sized wall of your gut. Once the gut wall is "leaky," lectins can damage your internal organs, your joint tissues, and, as some of my other research has shown, even be the source of autoimmune disorders such as rheumatoid arthritis, Hashimoto's thyroiditis, or diabetes mellitus, and coronary artery disease.

3. **Lectins are directly linked to weight gain.** Lectins, like WGA (*wheat germ agglutinin*, a protein found in whole wheat), stick to the insulin receptors on fat cells and constantly signal fat storage while blocking the hormone that controls your appetite, leptin. When leptin is blocked, your brain never gets the "message" you're full—so you just keep eating! Studies show conclusively that blocking this hormone actually causes weight gain.

Now, the good news is that most lectin-containing foods can be consumed when pressure cooked (for example in an Instant Pot, a tool that is becoming de rigueur for many home cooks); just keep in mind that a pressure cooker will not destroy gluten or break up a similar protein in oats.

Rule #7: Stop with the Sugar Already
One of the most concerning aspects of our modern diet is that many foods contain highly refined sugars and carbohydrates—but

most people don't even realize they're eating them. You have to understand how much sugar is really in food; it's not just the grams of sugar on a label! For instance, look at a bagel. While it says it has zero sugar on its label, the industrial milling process took what would have been a very complex starch that would otherwise have taken a long time to digest and turned it into rapidly available sugar; in fact, about 8 to 9 teaspoons' worth. White bread has a glycemic index of 100, which is higher than table sugar, because those individual starch molecules are instantly available as sugar. But, wait, you say, I don't see sugar listed on the label. You are right! Food labels were designed to hide the sugar content from you. There's an extra step you have to do to get an accurate sugar count: Take the total amount of carbs, subtract the fiber, and voila, there's how much sugar is in your food. For fun, you can divide that number by 4 to get the equivalent teaspoons of sugar in that serving. And remember, high-fructose corn syrup is in almost every prepackaged food, energy bar, and cookie. If you see the words "corn syrup," "brown rice syrup," "all natural syrup," or anything like that, just be aware that these are all forms of fructose, the ceramide-making mitochondrial energy buster that we want to avoid at all costs.

Luckily, when you want to indulge your sweet tooth, you have options—see the list of safer sugar substitutes on page 201, including one of my favorites, inulin, or allulose. Just please remember the golden rule with all these products: Overuse of them tricks the brain into thinking that real sugar is coming, and when it doesn't arrive, your brain can drive you to hunt for more and more food to satisfy that craving. Always use sugar substitutes, even healthy-seeming ones, in moderation. (And please nix the chemical sweeteners: If you've read any of my other books, you know that most artificial sweeteners, including sucralose, aspartame, and saccharine, kill gut bacteria. In fact, sucralose so disrupts bacteria in your gut that it promotes a pro-inflammatory state, so this is an absolute no-no.)[9] If it's hard to go cold turkey on any sweetening product, taper the amount you use over days and weeks—your taste buds will adjust over time.

Rule #8: Use Protein to Restore Flexibility, But Don't Overdo It

In my first book, *Dr. Gundry's Diet Evolution*, I recommended consuming animal protein as a primary source of calories in phase one, and as the program progressed, we gradually reduced animal protein to a small amount. I built the program that way because high-protein (whether plant or animal) diets can be useful temporarily to reset energy production. That's because digesting protein, particularly whole protein (let's say wild shrimp), requires a lot of energy. In fact, we lose about 30 percent of the calories in protein to digestion and heat generation. So, in a calorie-rich diet, burning a lot of the protein calories that you eat generates heat, and most people lose weight because of that effect. High-protein diets, like the modified Atkins, the carnivore diet, or the drinking man's diet (Robert Cameron, the author of the book on this diet, died at ninety-eight, by the way), work both by thermogenesis and by limiting mitochondrial energy sources to one substrate, hence no rush hour. You can take advantage of this benefit, if you want, as you start the program with the first meal of the day (break-fast) as a mono meal of high protein, as you will soon read.

So why not just stay on a high-protein diet forever? Mainly because it deprives your gut buddies of the fiber essential for the production of short-chain fatty acids, so critical to mitochondrial health, which plummet within days of starting a high-protein diet.[10] The production of SCFAs is *significantly* reduced in humans within days following a dietary change from a complex carbohydrate—rich, plant-based diet to an animal-based diet high in saturated fat and low in complex carbohydrates.[11] Moreover, a high-protein, low-carb diet suppresses butyrate production and creates other damaging compounds.[12] In addition, overconsumption of animal protein can cause *too* much H_2S production in the colon, which promotes colon cell injury.[13] Remember that Goldilocks effect—too much is not a good thing in this case.

I'm not vilifying animal-sourced protein; I just want you to have some perspective and make wise choices. If you eat animal protein, I suggest trying to include wild fish and wild shellfish in your diet; the smaller the fish, the better, like sardines, herring, and anchovies, as well as wild salmon, bivalves (clams, oysters, and the like), and other shellfish. Omega-3 eggs are another good bet for most people, but a number of my autoimmune patients sadly react to the proteins in both the whites and the yolks. When it comes to meat, please enjoy *smaller portions* (max 4 ounces) of the highest quality meat you can get, by which I mean 100 percent grass-fed and grass-finished or, in the case of poultry, pasture-raised. These meats will be free of the energy-disruptive antibiotics, hormones, and pesticides that we are attempting to avoid.

As for dairy products, devoted Paradox readers know the score here. Most cow's milk products in the US come from a type of cow that has a highly inflammatory type of milk protein called A1 casein. Please choose goat's or sheep's milk products (yogurt, cheese, milk, etc.) for this reason or cheeses from southern European (A2 casein) cows.

Now, rather than default to meat as a "must-have" protein source, consider that a gorilla or a horse has more muscles than you will ever have, and they only eat leaves and grasses! There is indeed protein available to you in a plant-rich meal. For example, there are 2 grams of protein in almost every serving of vegetables that you can name. I encourage you to try using low-lectin, healthy plant protein choices including pressure-cooked lentils (which have a whopping 18 grams of protein per cup, with about 15 grams of gut-buddy-friendly fiber) and hemp tofu and hemp protein hearts (hemp contains all the essential amino acids). You can also enjoy concentrated plant proteins in the form of nuts, which have anywhere from 4 to 9 grams of protein, including all of the essential amino acids, in a 1-ounce serving (1 ounce is about a handful). If you want to get more exotic, Barùkas nuts and Sacha Inchi seeds have the highest protein of any nut or seed. Three more plant-based protein sources are spirulina algae, flaxseed protein, and hemp protein powders.

Lectin-Mac Attack

There's no doubt you've come across the food industry's latest answer to a burger replacement which you may be tempted to use as a "good protein." It's the plant-based patties like the Impossible Burger and Beyond Burger. Both claim to taste, smell, and look like "the real thing." But should cows rejoice at the substitute for their meat? Not quite yet. Of course, the plant-based burger is an attempt to help protect animal welfare, but that doesn't necessarily mean they're healthy for you.

The Impossible Burger lists soy and potato proteins among other "natural flavors" as its main ingredients. The Beyond Burger lists pea and rice proteins. While the Beyond Burger is non-GMO, the Impossible Burger has faced criticism for containing GMOs and glyphosate, a deadly disruptor (see page 152). And the main ingredients of both burgers—pea and soy protein—are packed with lectins. The bottom line is that these are still heavily processed foods that irritate the gut and cause inflammation. As we used to ask at Loma Linda University Medical School, what "mystery meat" are we making today out of TVP (textured vegetable protein, high-pressure high heat–extruded soy)? My point: Eat whole foods please.

Rule #9: Don't Eat Frankenfoods Loaded with Frankenfats

The typical American diet is filled with highly processed, sugary, and fatty foods. We have known for some time that this type of diet is not only harmful to overall health by being pro-inflammatory, but it also dramatically decreases energy production,[14] and a common additive to junk food has been shown to alter our gut microbiota, and cause inflammation, especially in the colon.[15] And as if we needed more reasons, a diet high in bad fats, especially fried foods that contain polyunsaturated and trans fats (soybean oil, corn oil, etc.), destroys your ability to make hydrogen sulfide.[16] Hopefully what you read in Chapter 4 scared you away from the trans fats that are hiding in processed and fried foods. If you do consume them, I suggest getting your hands on some omega-3 fatty acids, either in the form of wild-caught salmon or good-quality supplements. Research shows that DHA and EPA can remodel the mitochondrial membrane by blocking the trans fats from getting incorporated in the membrane—in a sense, kicking those bad actors to the curb.[17]

One big reminder here: Please don't make the mistake that I'm suggesting you avoid all forms of fat! As you may know, I have long been a fan of olive oil, partially because of the extraordinary benefits of the polyphenols (and melatonin!) it contains. In fact, my favorite saying is "the only purpose of food is to get more olive oil into your mouth." Well, I now have another go-to oil: sesame oil. There is mounting research on its incredible benefits: One study has shown that just 2 tablespoons a day can drastically reduce high blood pressure.[18] It also blocks the effects of LPSs[19] (a big driver in insulin resistance) and electromagnetic fields (EMF) damage by being a superstrong antioxidant. So add some sesame oil in your daily food intake—it has a very high smoke point, making it a great choice for cooking.

It's Time for Chrono Consumption

Now that you have a better handle on what to eat and what not to eat to support your mitochondria and microbiome (M^2), let's turn to the C^2 part of the equation: chrono consumption. This is my approach to time-restricted feeding (a form of intermittent fasting), and it will help to reestablish your body's and your microbiome's natural circadian rhythms and train your metabolism to enter a fasted state each day.

This well-choreographed eating timetable involves timing your meals strategically to make the most of your body's rest and repair functions, while limiting the daylong rush hour hitting your mitochondria. Translation: You will increase the period between the last meal of one day and the first meal of the next. For some of you, this may be the most intimidating part of the program. After all, the dogma about breakfast being "the most important meal of the day" has been drilled into our heads for years, and many people struggle to start their day on an empty stomach.

But never fear: I'm going to make this easy for you. Now, I could ask you to wake up tomorrow and fast until noon (which, believe it or not, in six weeks will most likely be a breeze for you); but quite frankly, that would be the equivalent of adding a six-hour jet lag to your circadian clock and your microbiome's clock. And, if you've ever flown between continents, you know that you feel off-kilter and drained for days after arriving at your destination. Our goal here is to improve, not diminish, your energy. So, we're going to start slowly, with an eating window of twelve hours and gradually narrow that window to six to eight hours a day, while leaving a good three hours of not eating before bedtime. This gives your body, your mitochondria, your gut, and your poor addled brain much-needed time to rest, repair, and regenerate. And, as a reward and incentive, weekends are free to do whatever you want, within reason. Doesn't sound too bad, does it?

Now, here's the best part: Your first meal of the day, your "breakfast," is going to jump-start your energy production into high gear by making things really easy on your mitochondria. Welcome to the mono meal.

Mono Your Way into the Day

In addition to restricting your eating window, you're going to give your mitochondria another break by providing them with one fuel and one fuel only for the first meal of the day. Remember the effects of the mono diets we discussed in Chapter 4? While I don't recommend following them over an extended period of time, they are effective in the beginning because they reduce the mitochondrial traffic jam. We're going to borrow a page from their playbook with not a mono diet but a mono meal.

Your first meal of the day will be based on *one* macronutrient. Initially this meal will be made up of an almost pure protein, or almost pure carbohydrate source, and later, as the program progresses, you can choose mostly fat. Why wait on a pure fat meal? Because it's unlikely that you have the metabolic flexibility to burn fat right now. No cartwheels just yet. My experience with thousands of patients who plunge headlong into keto diets is that they usually crash and burn because their insulin levels are too high for their bodies to run on fat for fuel. But an all-protein or all-carb meal is still easy on your mitochondria and gives you all the energy you need.

Here's the best part: I don't care what macronutrient you choose and neither do your mitochondria. Dealer's choice! Carb day? Okay, how about a bowl of millet cereal with almond milk? How about a warm bowl of fonio (a tiny cousin of millet) prepared like oatmeal? Or a prebiotic shake? Or sweet potato hash browns? Time for a high-protein break-fast? As simple as a few scrambled egg whites (the whites are the protein part of the egg, the yolks are the fat), humanely raised ham or Canadian bacon, or some grass-fed, grass-finished jerky. Vegan options for protein include hemp protein powder shakes or a basil seed pudding (page 259) that puts chia puddings to shame! This first meal of the day is a little treat for your mitochondria—you are waking them up gently with a soft pop ballad rather than heavy metal. And here's more good news: You can mix it up! Egg whites one day, sorghum "oatmeal" the next, hemp shake the next, Canadian bacon or turkey sausage patties the next, or millet cereal every day. What kind of crazy eating program is this? I'll tell you what it is: It's one that works, is sustainable, and keeps you from getting stuck in a rut. Just remember, mono diets usually fail due to boredom. Not this time!

Once you make it to week 3, you can throw in fat break-fasts. My favorite is an avocado, cut in half, the pit replaced with two egg yolks and popped into the toaster oven or broiler, then drizzled with olive oil and sprinkled with salt and pepper. Yummy! Or what about a nice big hunk of triple cream Brie from France? Vegans, how about a pitted olive–stuffed avocado drizzled with olive oil? There are plenty of satisfying options, no matter which mono you choose.

Water Fasting Is Not the Fastest Route to Energy Production

With all this talk of limiting eating windows, you might be tempted to simply do a full-on fasting program instead, where only water is consumed for several days (or longer). While there are many benefits to all forms of fasting (see page 126), I do not recommend a traditional water fast as a part of this program. Here's the thing: When you stop eating, you also stop feeding your microbiome. Yes, I'm all for starving off the bad guys, but we want to give the good guys a lift. Fasting won't easily do that. Moreover, most people aren't easily able to use stored fat as a fuel because they are contending with chronically high insulin levels; so, when they fast, their energy disappears. Not exactly what we're looking for, right? Not to mention, if you're overweight and begin a fasting regimen, your body lets go of the heavy metals and environmental toxins that are stored in body fat. Rapid weight loss releases massive amounts of these toxins, which cannot be safely detoxified by our liver. And you can guess what toxins do to your mitochondria! On the Energy Paradox Program's eating schedule, you'll get all the benefits of fasting without the downsides.

The six-week Energy Paradox Program is incremental, so each week will break down like this: Monday through Friday you will delay your break-fast by one hour and you will try to finish your last meal by 7 p.m. In other words, if you have break-fast at 7 a.m. on Monday, you'll have break-fast at 8 a.m. on Tuesday, 9 a.m. on Wednesday, and so on, finishing eating by 7 p.m. every day. Then, each successive week will restart the same pattern, delaying your first meal of the week by another hour. By week 6, you will have arrived at your goal of starting break-fast at noon and limiting your total eating window to seven hours (12 p.m. to 7 p.m.). And remember, your break-fast will be your choice of a mono meal—protein, carb, and after two weeks, fat if you want.

Come the weekend, you may be more flexible, within reason; have breakfast when you like, and create your plate as you like, still following the Dos and Don'ts and eating the approved foods listed on pages 194 to 204. The idea isn't to binge on donuts, but simply to allow yourself the flexibility to enjoy weekend meals with family and friends if you choose.

It looks like this:

WEEK	Monday Breakfast	Tuesday Breakfast	Wednesday Breakfast	Thursday Breakfast	Friday Breakfast
1	7 A.M.	8 A.M.	9 A.M.	10 A.M.	11 A.M.
2	8 A.M.	9 A.M.	10 A.M.	11 A.M.	12 P.M.
3	9 A.M.	10 A.M.	11 A.M.	12 P.M.	12 P.M.
4	10 A.M.	11 A.M.	12 P.M.	12 P.M.	12 P.M.
5	11 A.M.	11 A.M.	12 P.M.	12 P.M.	12 P.M.
6	12 P.M.	12 P.M.	12 P.M.	12 P.M.	12 P.M.

Okay, you may be asking, why do we nearly reset the clock at the beginning of each week and start just one hour later than the previous week's first meal? The reason for this staggered approach in which you push break-fast back gradually over five days, take a break over the weekend, and then start the same routine over, is that much like with a fitness regimen, we are slowly training your body to adhere to a new routine. Your circadian clocks and your mitochondria are gaining strength and flexibility, similar to your muscles, adding a little more time and effort each day. This has proved to be a very reliable way to *gradually* condition your metabolism, training it without shocking it by going "too hard, too fast." Plus, I've noticed, having done this for twenty years with myself and with my patients, that having freedom on the weekends is very useful to staying the course. In fact, in successful four- and six-hour eating window studies in humans, taking the weekend off really helped with compliance and didn't affect the participants becoming metabolically flexible.[20]

At the end of the sixth week, you will be cruising along an eight-hour eating window for five days a week. Not only will your metabolism be trained to shift into fat-burning easily, and happily creating ketones that switch on important cleanup, repair, and regenerative processes throughout your body, but the habit of delaying your first meal of the day will be well established. You won't be fighting it or even thinking about it anymore. And I assure you, noticeably improved energy levels will be a happy outcome of this hard work.

In fact, after the six weeks are up, you may find it pretty effortless to keep up this routine. Gaining metabolic flexibility is a gift that allows you to eat when you want to and enjoy more energy all the time. My hope for you is that, unlike with some diets and programs, you don't go back to your old routine. Make this schedule your new normal, and your mitochondria, your circadian rhythms, and your microbiome will thank you. And those of you who aced this program and want to kick things up a notch, I've got you covered. You can join me in eating only one meal a day, the so-called EOMAD program, which I will cover in more detail shortly (see page 192).

What to Drink

Limiting your food eating window doesn't mean depriving you of hydration. You should always have plenty of water or other liquids, and no, black coffee or tea doesn't dehydrate you. Here are a few other liquid options that are Energy Paradox–approved.

Hydrogen water: If you want to up your energy game, you can drink water with added hydrogen molecules. There are now over 1,500 published studies on the gasomessenger hydrogen (H_2) and the benefits of drinking hydrogen water (which is what it sounds like: hydrogen dissolved into water), and many of them show how it can fight fatigue.[21] Since hydrogen is the smallest molecule, it diffuses instantly through your gut wall. Hydrogen water is available in cans, although it is far more convenient to dissolve hydrogen tablets in water and drink it once a day. It is fairly pricey, so if you are cost-conscious, fresh filtered water still gets the job done.

Caffeine: Feel free to indulge your morning caffeine intake and have tea—green, black, or herbal—and black coffee. Remember, if you add anything to your coffee or tea, including cream or butter, you officially broke your overnight fast. Okay, not quite ready to give up the creamer? Try unsweetened almond, hemp, coconut, pistachio, or macadamia milk, but, honestly, try to limit them. I'll have more to say about MCT oil shortly. Good news: Approved no-calorie sweeteners or prebiotics (which, by definition, you cannot digest) do not count against you in terms of breaking a fast.

Alcohol: Four to six ounces of organic or biodynamic red wine or champagne or one ounce of dark spirits is allowed during dinner.

Don't "Skip Out" on Meal Skipping

I'm going to be straight with you: When you first start this program, it's very likely that you will be hungry. I always tell my patients to embrace their hunger, not hide from it or panic about it, but I'm also a realist. I understand that in the beginning of this program, some people will struggle with some discomfort. Especially in the first week or so, you may find it difficult to keep pushing back breakfast later and later. If you feel this way, it's because your body is not yet metabolically flexible enough to make these changes.

The end goal here is to stick with the program long enough to reap its benefits, so if you are really struggling, I say, take it easy and make it work for you. For instance, let's say you did great on Monday and Tuesday, but Wednesday rolls around and you don't feel like you have the energy you need to make it to 9 a.m. to eat. If you had gotten to 8 a.m. in good shape, just stay there, or try for 8:30. Next week, set a new goal.

If you're dealing with hunger pangs, prebiotic fiber is a great way to keep hunger at bay. Just mix a scoop in some water and drink up. It has no calories for you, as you can't digest it, but your gut buddies can, and they'll send a message to your brain that they're content and you don't need to give them more food! Plus, they'll get right to work producing butyrate, that incredible mitochondrial fuel and healer.

If you want to follow your timetable with a little less discomfort, or you can't make it to the break-fast, you can also pick up some MCT (medium-chain triglyceride) oil, sometimes called liquid coconut oil, available in many grocery stores. It can be easily and rapidly converted into ketones in your liver, and it's tasteless and flavorless. When all else fails, take about 1 teaspoon to 1 tablespoon three times a day for the first few days, and you'll get through those sinking spells. A word of warning, especially for my female readers, whose stomachs seem to be more sensitive to it than men: Use MCT sparingly. If you take too much when you're just starting out, you will be spending a lot of your energy on trips to the bathroom—and flushing some gut buddies down the drain as well. If you're trying to get to the point of making your own ketones, you can take a few capsules or a scoop of preformed ketones, in the form of ketone salts or esters, which will give you a small but rapidly acting dose of the real thing (more on this on page 268).

Another trick is to keep a handful of nuts nearby, and whenever a hunger pang feels unbearable, eat a few nuts. Salted nuts are best. When we're actively losing weight, we urinate a lot, and we lose salt. Research shows that it's beneficial to increase your salt intake when you first start limiting your eating window, and doing so will also help prevent cravings.[22] So don't be afraid of a little salt—it's not the enemy that everybody thinks it is. Just make sure it's iodized sea salt, not the pink stuff (see page 92).

No matter what, go easy on yourself—it is perfectly normal to experience cravings and feel tired at first. It takes some time to starve out the bad bugs and shut down their chatter. The more you can ride out the discomfort, the faster they'll leave!

Resetting the Clock Versus Beating the Clock

The average American eats all day long. Unlike the common perception that we sit down to three square meals a day with maybe a couple of snacks in between, few of us actually sit down to proper meals anymore. Research shows that most people eat for sixteen hours a day. We're busy, on the move, grabbing a quick bite here and there, any time of day or night. We've become a land of munchers, grazers, and mini-meal eaters.

So if you can narrow your eating window to just twelve hours as a starting off point, and then slowly compress that window down to six to eight hours a day, you can reach an eating window you can live with, literally and figuratively. Now remember, you are going to get there gradually. This is the same approach I use (to great success) in my practice, and so many of my patients are just like you.

In fact, the vast majority of people I initially see in my clinics are insulin resistant and metabolically inflexible. It's an important point to understand that if you have an elevated insulin level, it is very difficult to jump right into time-restricted eating, because it's impossible for the body to mobilize free fatty acids from fat stores when it's been running on sugar for so long. Why fight biology? When you're metabolically inflexible you simply *can't get into ketosis*, much less use free fatty acids as a fuel source. That's right, you *can't*. All of the willpower in the world will not get your body to make ketones. On top of that, if you try to bite the bullet and force your body into ketosis, you will feel terrible: low energy, grouchy, "hangry." You will suffer the "keto flu" or "Atkins blues." Most of my new patients have never had their fasting insulin level measured before walking into my clinics, and have stories of failed attempts at intermittent fasting, a keto diet, or just cutting calories drastically. They blame themselves, but the reality is they never had a chance of success—they didn't have the mitochondrial flexibility to use free fatty acids as a fuel or the ability to liberate free fatty acids from their fat cells that they could then make into ketones in their liver. They were stuck on a dead-end street of using sugar for poor energy production. Thus, when you start removing all the sugars, starches, and junk from your diet, you actually go through sugar withdrawal because your mitochondria can't use fat for fuel. But, with my staggered plan, you will taper off sugar slowly so it's not a sudden plunge—I'll walk you down the mountain, rather than throw you off a cliff.

Now maybe you're thinking, "Listen, I'm not one of your usual patients, Dr. G. I eat healthy, organic food. But I'm still exhausted. What about me?" A few things: Remember those deadly disrupters from Chapter 6? We need to get rid of them, or at least neutralize their effects. Second, most of you "healthy eaters" are consuming a smorgasbord of lectin-rich foods that are destroying your gut wall, producing inflammation. Out they go on this program. Finally, remember those mice who ate healthy rat chow but were the all-day munchers? They had no metabolic flexibility compared to the mice with compressed eating windows. If you're eating healthily, but constantly, you're still setting yourself up for an energy drain. Last, some of my self-described "healthiest eaters" are also fruit-aholics, and have absolutely overwhelmed their livers and mito-chondria with energy-robbing fructose.[23,24]

Now here's the great news: Even after your first baby steps on the program you will start to notice a real difference in your energy levels and overall well-being, because both microbiome and mito-chondrial changes occur quickly when you make dietary changes. And feeling better will help you stay motivated to keep going. Remember, you don't have to be perfect. The most important thing is to "do what you can, with what you've got, wherever you are."

Every now and then, I have patients who cannot or will not give up breakfast at, well, breakfast time. They have to start off the day by eating something, or else! Usually, the tricks I've shared here get them over the hump. But if all else fails, there is one more workaround.

Eat, Pause, Eat

If you truly cannot start your day without eating something, I recommend following a Ramadan-style fast. As we discussed on page 134, research shows that those who fast during Ramadan receive the same benefits as those who employ time-controlled eating. During the month of Ramadan, practitioners eat a small meal before sunrise and then don't eat or drink until after sunset, when they eat their main meal. By having a twelve-hour non-eating window during the day, followed by an approximate eight-hour non-eating window during sleep, they are essentially fasting twenty hours per day.

Why try this option? Giving up breakfast is tough for a lot of people who structure their day around a morning meal. Often, in a normal workday, lunch may just get in the way, so many people opt to eat breakfast and skip lunch. If you are in this camp, or if you have trouble on the chrono consumption path, and I mean this sincerely, I don't want to lose you and your mitochondria to the struggle. Before you give up, try eating a mono break-fast (preferably high protein) and then skip lunch and wait for dinner for your last meal. And who knows, once you become metabolically flexible, you might feel ready to start delaying break-fast later and later.

If you've advanced on the chrono consumption path and want to keep going during the weekends, why not add this eat, pause, eat option? This is actually what I do almost every weekend, all year long.

Turbo Boost Energy Paradox Program: EOMAD

For those readers who are doing great after six weeks and are looking for a new challenge, I recommend advancing to an EOMAD phase: eat one meal a day. I know this strategy works because I've been doing it for the last eighteen years. I can tell you firsthand, its workable, doable, and sustainable. When my patients try this technique, their IGF-1 levels plummet, as does their HbA1c, both huge benefits in the longevity game. I'm convinced that drastically reducing the amount of time and energy your body must devote to digestion and easing the gridlock of mitochondrial rush hour is one of the best things we can do for our health.

If you want to give it a try, I suggest doing so after the six-week marker, when at week 7 you eat your first meal at 1 p.m., and quit eating at 7 p.m. At week 8, your first meal will start at 2 p.m., and at week 9, your first meal will start at 3 p.m. You are now at a four-hour eating window; you can stop anytime, but, hey, push through two more weeks and you've reached the two-hour EOMAD.

And, by the way, one of the best effects of this EOMAD is all that extra free time you have by not eating. We laugh at my office, as my "lunch hour" is spent on podcasts or writing, not eating. Incredibly liberating! Oh, by the way, I'm never hungry. I just remember to give my gut buddies their fair share when I do EOMAD. That way they and I don't GOMAD!

What about Calorie Counting and "Macros"?

Unlike a lot of popular diets, you don't have to worry about counting calories or macronutrients on the Energy Paradox Program. Calorie counts are pretty meaningless, particularly if a lot of those calories are being eaten by your gut buddies, and frankly, I'm not concerned with your ratio of protein, fat, and carbohydrates. And you don't need to restrict calories for this to work. In fact, time-controlled eating works to fix metabolic flexibility better than calorie restriction.[25] Energy production depends on limiting your eating window and your mitochondrial fuel choices, not limiting calories or macros. In the end, if I can get you to both limit the amount of time you're eating and make sure that some of the foods you're eating also feed your gut buddies, that's what's going to help you feel the difference in your energy (and, most of the time, see it on the scale and feel it in how your clothes fit).

The Energy Paradox Program Food Lists

Okay, dear reader, here it is: the lists you've been waiting for. The following "yes" and "no" lists make up the backbone of the Energy Paradox Program. These lists of foods should be considered complementary to the Do and Don'ts rules you read earlier, and are great resources for quick and easy reference. As always, you can find this information online as well at www.DrGundry.com, where you can access a downloadable PDF.

Energy-Boosting Foods

Cruciferous Vegetables

arugula	kimchi
bok choy	kohlrabi
broccoli	napa cabbage
Brussels sprouts	radicchio
cabbage (green and red)	sauerkraut (raw)
cauliflower	Swiss chard
collards	watercress
kale	

Other Vegetables

artichokes	chives
asparagus	daikon radish
bamboo shoots	fiddlehead ferns
beets (raw)	garlic
carrot greens	garlic scapes
carrots (raw)	ginger
celery	hearts of palm
chicory	horseradish

Jerusalem artichokes (sunchokes)

leeks

lemongrass

mushrooms

nopales (cactus; available online)

okra

onions

parsnips

puntarella

radishes

rutabaga

scallions

shallots

water chestnuts

Leafy Greens

algae

basil

butter lettuce

cilantro

dandelion greens

endive

escarole

fennel

mesclun (baby greens)

mint

mizuna

mustard greens

parsley

perilla

purslane

red and green leaf lettuces

romaine lettuce

sea vegetables

seaweed

spinach

Fruits That Act like Fats

Avocado (up to a whole one per day)   Olives, all types

Oils

algae oil (Thrive culinary brand)

avocado oil

black seed oil

canola oil (non-GMO, organic only!)

coconut oil

cod liver oil (the lemon and orange
    flavors have no fish taste)

macadamia oil

MCT oil

olive oil (extra virgin)

perilla oil

pistachio oil

red palm oil

rice bran oil

sesame oil (plain and toasted)

walnut oil

Nuts and Seeds (1/2 cup per day)

almonds (only blanched or Marcona)

Barùkas nuts

Brazil nuts (in limited amounts, about 3 a day for selenium)

chestnuts

coconut (not coconut water)

coconut milk (unsweetened dairy substitute)

coconut milk/cream (unsweetened, full-fat, canned)

flaxseeds

hazelnuts

hemp protein powder

hemp seeds

macadamia nuts

Milkadamia creamer (unsweetened)

nut butters (if almond butter, preferably made with peeled almonds, as almond skins contain lectins)

pecans

pili nuts

pine nuts

pistachios

psyllium seeds

Sacha Inchi seeds

sesame seeds

tahini (sesame paste)

walnuts

Energy Bars (limit to one per day, please)

Adapt Bars: Coconut and Chocolate

B-Up (made by Yup): Chocolate Mint, Chocolate Chip Cookie Dough, Sugar Cookie

GundryMD Bars

Keto Bars: Almond Butter Brownie, Salted Caramel, Lemon Poppyseed, Chocolate Chip Cookie Dough

MariGold Bars: ChocoNut, Pure Joy, Espresso, Ginger Coconut

Primal Kitchen Bars: Almond Spice and Coconut Lime

Quest Bars: Lemon Cream Pie, Banana Nut, Strawberry Cheesecake, Cinnamon Roll, Double Chocolate Chunk, Maple Waffle, Mocha Chocolate Chip, Peppermint Bark, Chocolate Sprinkled Doughnut, Cinnamon Roll

Rowdy Bars: Keto Chocolaty Cookie Dough

Stoka: Vanilla Almond and Coco Almond

Processed Resistant Starches (can be eaten every day in limited quantities)

(Note: people with diabetes or prediabetes should consume only once a week on average)

Barely Bread's bread and bagels (only those without raisins)

Cappello's fettucine and other pasta

California Country Gal Sandwich Bread

Egg Thins by Crepini

Julian Bakery Paleo Wraps (made with coconut flour), Paleo Thin Bread Almond Bread, Sandwich Bread, Coconut Bread

Mikey's Original and Toasted Onion English Muffins

Positively Plantain tortillas

Real Coconut Coconut and Cassava Flour Tortillas and Chips

Siete brand chips (be careful here—a couple of my canaries react to the small amount of chia seeds in the chips) and tortillas (only those made with cassava and coconut flour or almond flour)

Simple Mills Almond Flour Crackers

sorghum pasta

SRSLY sourdough non-lectin bread and rice-free sourdough rolls

Terra Cassava, Taro, and Plantain Chips

Thrive Market Organic Coconut Flakes

Trader Joe's Jicama Wraps

Trader Joe's Plantain Chips

Resistant Starches (in moderation)

(Note: people with diabetes and prediabetes should initially limit these foods)

baobab fruit

cassava (tapioca)

celery root (celeriac)

glucomannan (konjac root)

green bananas

green mango

green papaya

green plantains

jicama

millet

parsnips

persimmon

rutabaga

sorghum

sweet potatoes or yams

taro root

tiger nuts

turnips

yucca

"Foodles" (acceptable "noodles")

Cassava pastas

Edison Grainery sorghum pasta

GundryMD's Pasta

Jovial cassava pastas

Kanten Pasta

kelp noodles

konjac noodles

millet pasta (Bgreen Food brand, all types except angel hair pasta)

Miracle Noodles

Miracle Rice

Natural Heaven Hearts of Palm Spaghetti and Lasagna

Palmini Hearts of Palm Noodles

shirataki noodles

Slim Pasta

Sweet Potato Pasta elbow macaroni

Trader Joe's Cauliflower Gnocchi

Seafood (any wild-caught, 4 ounces per day)

Alaskan salmon

anchovies

calamari/squid

clams

cod

crab

freshwater bass

halibut

Hawaiian fish, including mahi-mahi, ono, and opah

lobster

mussels

oysters

sardines

scallops

shrimp (wild only)

tuna (canned)

whitefish

Pastured Poultry (4 ounces per day)

chicken

duck

game birds (pheasant, grouse, dove, quail)

goose

ostrich

pastured or omega-3 eggs (up to 4 daily)

turkey

Meat (100 percent grass-fed and grass-finished, 4 ounces per day)

beef

bison

boar

elk

grass-fed jerky (low-sugar versions)

lamb

pork (humanely raised, including prosciutto, Iberico ham, 5J ham), Canadian bacon, ham

venison

wild game

Plant-Based Proteins and "Meats"

hemp tofu

Hilary's Root Veggie Burger

Kelp Jerky

pressure-cooked lentils and other legumes (canned, such as Eden or Jovial brand) or dried, soaked†, then pressure cooked (use an Instant Pot)

Quorn products: only Meatless Pieces, Meatless Grounds, Meatless Steak-Style Strips, Meatless Fillets, Meatless Roast (avoid all others, as they contain lectins/gluten)

Fruits (limit to one small serving on weekends and only when that fruit is in season)

(Best options are pomegranate and passion fruit seeds, followed by raspberries, blackberries, strawberries, then blueberries)

apples

apricots

blackberries

blueberries

cherries

citrus (no juices)

crispy pears (Anjou, Bosc, Comice)

kiwis

nectarines

passion fruit

peaches

plums

pomegranates

raspberries

strawberries

---

† Soaking and pressure cooking instructions for lentils and legumes are easily found online.

Dairy Products and Replacements
(limit to 1 ounce cheese or 4 ounces yogurt per day)

A2 casein milk

buffalo butter (available at Trader Joe's)

buffalo mozzarella (Italian)

cheeses from Switzerland

coconut yogurt (plain)

French/Italian butter

French/Italian cheese

ghee (grass-fed)

goat's and sheep's milk kefir (plain)

goat's milk cheese

goat's milk creamer

goat's milk yogurt (plain)

Kite Hill Cream Cheese Alternative

Kite Hill (plant-based) yogurts

Kite Hill ricotta (almond-based)

Lavva (plant-based) yogurt

organic cream cheese

organic heavy cream

organic sour cream

Parmigiano-Reggiano

sheep's milk cheese

sheep's milk yogurt (plain)

whey protein powder (grass-fed cow, goat, sheep)

Herbs, Seasonings, and Condiments

avocado mayonnaise

coconut aminos

fish sauce (no sugar added)

herbs and spices (all except chile flakes)

miso

mustard

nutritional yeast

sea salt (ideally iodized)

tahini

vanilla extract (pure)

vinegars (any without added sugar)

wasabi

Flours

almond (blanched)

arrowroot

cassava

chestnut

coconut

coffee fruit

grape seed

green banana

hazelnut

millet

sesame (and seeds)

sorghum flour

sweet potato

tiger nut

Sweeteners

allulose (look for non-GMO)

erythritol (Swerve is my favorite, as it also contains oligosaccharides)

inulin (Just Like Sugar is a great brand)

local honey and/or manuka honey (very limited!)

monkfruit; also known as luo han guo (Lakanto brand is good)

stevia (SweetLeaf is my favorite)

xylitol

yacón (Sunfood Sweet Yacon Syrup is available on Amazon)

Chocolate and Frozen Desserts

coconut milk dairy-free frozen desserts (the So Delicious blue label, which contains only 1 gram of sugar)

dark chocolate, unsweetened, 72% or greater (1 ounce per day)

Enlightened Ice Cream

Keto Ice Cream: Chocolate, Mint Chip, Sea Salt Caramel

Killer Creamery Ice Cream: Chilla in Vanilla, Caramels Back, No Judge Mint

Mammoth Creameries: Vanilla Bean

nonalkalized cocoa powder

Rebel Creamery Ice Cream: Butter Pecan, Raspberry, Salted Caramel, Strawberry, and Vanilla

Simple Truth Ice Cream: Butter Pecan and Chocolate Chip

Beverages

Champagne (6 ounces per day)

coffee

dark spirits (1 ounce per day)

hydrogen water

KeVita brand low-sugar kombucha (such as coconut and coconut Mojito)

Pellegrino or Panna water

red wine (6 ounces per day)

tea (all types)

The "No, Thank You" List of Lectin-Containing Foods

Refined, Starchy Foods

bread

cereal

cookies

crackers

pasta

pastries

potato chips

potatoes

rice

tortillas

wheat flour

Grains, Sprouted Grains, Pseudo-Grains, and Grasses

barley (cannot pressure cook)

barley grass

brown rice

buckwheat

bulgur

corn

corn products

corn syrup

einkorn

kamut

kasha

oats (cannot pressure cook)

popcorn

quinoa

rye (cannot pressure cook)

spelt

wheat

wheat (cannot pressure cook; pressure cooking does not remove lectins from any form of wheat)

wheatgrass

white rice (except pressure-cooked white basmati rice from India[†])

wild rice

Sugar and Sweeteners

agave

coconut sugar

diet drinks

granulated sugar (even organic cane sugar)

maltodextrin

NutraSweet (aspartame)

Splenda (sucralose)

Sweet One from Sunett (acesulfame-K)

Sweet'n Low (saccharin)

---

† The Indian variety of white basmati rice is high-resistant starch; the American variety not.

Vegetables

beans* (all, including sprouts)	peas
chickpeas* (including as hummus)	soy
edamame	soy protein
green beans	sugar snap peas
legumes*	textured vegetable protein (TVP)
lentils* (all)	tofu
pea protein	

Allowable only if they are properly prepared in a pressure cooker.

Nuts and Seeds

almonds with peels	peanuts
cashews	pumpkin seeds
chia seeds	sunflower seeds

Fruits (some called vegetables)

bell peppers	pumpkin
chiles	squash (any kind)
cucumbers	tomatillos
eggplant	tomatoes
goji berries	zucchini
melons (any kind)	

Milk Products That Contain A1 Casein

butter (even grass-fed), unless from A2 cows, sheep, or goats	ice cream
	kefir
cheese	milk
cottage cheese	ricotta
frozen yogurt	yogurt (including Greek yogurt)

Oils

canola (most is GMO)	peanut
corn	safflower
cottonseed	soy
grape-seed	sunflower
partially hydrogenated oils	vegetable

Herbs and Seasonings

ketchup	soy sauce
mayonnaise (except avocado mayonnaise)	steak sauce
	Worcestershire sauce
red chile flakes	

So there you have it: an eating program that heals your gut, nourishes your gut buddies, and ensures your mitochondria get what they need to maximize energy production. Now it's time to turn to the other choices you make every day that impact your get-up-and-go. It's time to take a hard look at your overall lifestyle and identify—and eliminate—the hidden sources of energy drain.

Troubleshooting

Q: *What if I have to attend a late dinner? What do I do the next day?*

First of all, I get it. Life happens. Maybe you have an important dinner meeting that starts at 8 and you don't finish the meal until 9 or 10. The next morning, just pick up where you left off—if you have your eating window down to ten hours, try to push your breakfast until noon. Once you fall off the horse, as I tell all my patients, just get right back on. One day is not going to make that big a difference.

Q: *I'm having a hard time getting started with the program. Do you have any suggestions for dealing with cravings and hunger?*

Well, first of all, cravings for junk foods are completely normal. Remember, your bad gut bugs are behind the scenes, pulling the strings on your desire for these foods, and it takes a little while to starve them out. Believe me, I know their messages are compelling. It's kind of like Odysseus and the Sirens' song. You need to be lashed to the mast for a few days! One way to help you stay on track is to enlist your support system—your significant other, your friend, coworker, whomever—for help. Ask them to remind you of all the reasons you're doing this program and promise them you won't get mad when they help you stay accountable! If all else fails, consider me your crew—you can always go back to this book and read about how much better you'll feel once you change up your nutrition. Give it three days: The bad guys will take off, and you will start to crave the foods that feed your gut buddies.

In my exam room, I've got not only a big poster of Yoda, but also several Yoda dolls, and one of our mottos is "Try not. Do or do not. There is no try." As you start break-fast later and later, and the hunger strikes, embrace it. As I assure all my patients: You will not starve to death.

Q: *How do I keep this up on a holiday?*

One of the huge benefits of this plan is the built-in "time off" for good behavior. Luckily, many holidays happen over a three-day weekend, so don't be afraid to start the week plan off on Tuesday instead of Monday. But do remember, I and others have so many YouTube or Instagram posts on how to make great holiday meals that are Energy Paradox compliant, that you don't need to go off the rails to enjoy yourself.

Q: *How do I get my family on board?*

First and foremost, this program is about getting your energy back. And the more energy you have, the more your family will want whatever it is that you're having (with a nod to *When Harry Met Sally*). And, like I said above, make your family members your crew who will keep you responsible. I can't tell you the number of kids who read their mother or father (or both) the riot act when they aren't eating approved "yes" foods.

Q: *I have to travel for work. How can I stay on track with the plan, especially when I'm in a different time zone?*

Before COVID-19, I traveled extensively, lecturing, presenting my work at international conferences, and studying long-lived, vigorously healthy people around the world. The reality is that you can enjoy eating on this program anywhere. Just remember that your circadian clock and your microbiome's clocks will be disrupted when you travel across time zones. Expose yourself to bright light and stay up "late" the day arriving so you can go to bed at the "new" proper time. Moreover, taking a dose of probiotics and prebiotics for several days after arrival helps to reset the microbiome clock. Finally, consider supplementing with 3 to 5 mg timed-release melatonin for a few days.

Q: *My work keeps me on a late schedule—I often don't get home until 7 or 8 p.m.—how can I do this?*

I worked the night shift as a scrub tech all through college, so I understand the crazy hours. Studies in mice (who are nighttime eaters) have found that when a mouse's eating window is shortened, they are protected from obesity and diabetes even when fed a high-fat/high-sugar diet.[26] Other research has shown that six hours of restricted eating is as effective as a very tight four-hour window of eating for weight loss.[27] If you eat late, start the program at twelve hours from your last meal the night before and advance the breakfast by one hour a day each day. Your break-fast may begin at 3 p.m.!

CHAPTER 8

THE ENERGY PARADOX LIFESTYLE

The pulse of the modern world and the conveniences that come with it—temperature control that either cools us down on a blazing hot day or warms us up on a biting cold morning, electricity that illuminates our homes when the sun goes down, cars that take us from point A to point B in minutes—have certainly improved our lives in innumerable ways. But these great innovations that make life *easier* actually make it *harder* for our bodies to function optimally. The human body has not only been designed to endure challenge, but to thrive on it. Our physiology requires moderate levels of biological and environmental discomfort to function at its best, and it is up to us to see to it that our bodies find the challenge they crave.

The choices we make every day can add up to a collective energy boost or, conversely, an energy drain. I've organized these lifestyle factors into six categories that I call the "Six Ss": Sweat, Sunlight, Shutdown Mode, Sleep, Sensory Challenges, and Stress Management.

It's not news that today we are more physically inactive than at any point in human history, and that our sedentary lifestyles are negatively impacting our health, making us more prone to developing obesity and other metabolic diseases. The same modern conveniences that have made life more enjoyable have also made it all too easy to sit still for prolonged periods of time. While it may seem like "conserving" energy would prevent us from feeling drained, in reality, the opposite is true: You need to use energy to make energy.

Sweat: It Takes Energy to Make Energy

Our bodies are designed for movement. You may recall the study on the super-fit and healthy Hadza tribe from Chapter 1. While the Hadzas' hunter-gatherer lifestyle makes them considerably more active than the average American office worker, even when the Hadzas are "at rest," they are not fully sedentary. For example, something as simple as sitting down and standing up is vastly more dynamic for them: They squat or, rather, sit on their haunches. As you are reading this paragraph, try getting out of your comfy seat and squatting on your haunches—you will feel the muscles in the backs of your legs and your glutes light up. Getting up and down fully to the ground many times over as part of daily life requires constant engagement of large muscles and uses the full range of motion of the joints. This steady movement uses energy, keeps our metabolic fires burning, and promotes mitochondrial efficiency.

Research shows that any type of sustained movement that keeps your body active and muscles engaged can be considered a cardiovascular activity. In fact, there is strong research showing that even low-level movement, such as fidgeting—tapping of the pen or tapping of feet—appears to help keep systems using energy more efficiently and can burn up to 300 to 350 more calories a day.[1] In today's culture so many people have internalized the idea that "fitness" can only be achieved through a special (and usually expensive) type of activity or class—but the human body was not designed to sit for ten hours a day and then get up and do Zumba for forty-five minutes. I believe we need to rethink our idea of exercise and instead of seeking out elaborate routines, simply emulate the physical activity of the Hadza tribe and *move more* to keep our energy system in good working order. Anytime you use the muscles in your body, even if it is just doing housework or standing at an upright desk, you burn glucose, then stored glycogen, and eventually (if you're not eating carbs while at your standing desk), your mitochondria shift to burning fatty acids. If you move your body more vigorously (like that Zumba class), you will start to produce and burn ketones.

This is metabolic flexibility in a nutshell, and regular movement helps keep your mitochondrial fires burning. The great news is that it's never too late to get moving: Research shows that movement and exercise can restore diminished mitochondrial function.[2] Plus, there's evidence that the benefits we reap from exercise in mitochondrial function and regeneration endure with time as we age.[3] Exercise also helps keep the body sensitive to insulin, and therefore has been proved to be protective against insulin resistance and diabetes.

Another great chain reaction that happens in your body when you engage your muscles—whether at a low or high intensity—is that newly discovered signaling molecules called *myokines* are produced, and they influence just about every organ system, including the brain. In fact, research shows that myokines may be the reason why regular exercise boosts cognitive health. As I have covered in my book *The Longevity Paradox*, exercise is correlated with less brain fog, reduced anxiety, and decreased risk of neurodegeneration, including Alzheimer's and dementia. In addition to benefiting your brain, exercise-induced myokines also support your energy-making mitochondria by stimulating mitogenesis, or the birth of new mitochondria.[4,5] These guys also boost your brainpower, help to stave off neurodegeneration, and allow you to get a good night's sleep (just try to finish up sixty to ninety minutes before bed to avoid overstimulation).

It's clear that moving your body is a nonnegotiable—the benefits are just too significant to pass up. The question is: How can we create an exercise program that works for you? If you're reading this book, chances are you don't have a ton of extra time for a new exercise routine—you're already overscheduled and exhausted. So let's work on meeting you where you are now, and consider how you can get the most gain with the least investment of pain (and time).

Exercise Snacking

Contrary to what you may think, you don't need to exercise for forty-five minutes or more to reap the benefits of movement. In fact, studies show that three ten-minute sessions of exercise scattered throughout the day offers at least the same, and perhaps even more, benefit as thirty minutes of continuous exercise.[6,7] The overall goal is to move continuously *throughout* the day, with "bursts" of vigorous movement included here and there that condition your metabolism to become more flexible.

In the Energy Paradox Program, I call these short sessions "snacks"; they are quick, easy forms of exercise that can be done anywhere, anytime. If you're new to exercise, even something as simple as going for a ten-minute walk is a great place to begin because walking is embedded in our evolutionary design—our genes expect us to walk! A daily walk can help kick-start energy production, improve metabolism, slash the risk of diabetes,[8] and help boost mental clarity. In fact, a 2016 study found that a ten-minute after-dinner stroll dramatically lowers blood sugars[9]; and you know what delaying that hit of sugar can do for your energy production. I love to take an evening stroll with my wife, Penny, and our dogs, who are always eager to get outside. (I often tell my patients that getting a dog is a great investment in their long-term health—studies show dog owners live longer than non–dog owners!)[10]

If possible, try to take your daily walks up and down hills to stress more muscles and reap even greater benefits. If you don't live in an area where that's a viable option, you can get the same benefits indoors. Does your home or workplace have a set of stairs? Studies show that as little as one minute of briskly walking up and down stairs improves mitochondrial function, while five or ten minutes offers even greater benefits.[11,12]

Step It Up with Fasted Exercise

While talking a walk after dinner is great, I also recommend getting in some movement in the morning. As we discussed in Chapter 6, you reap even more benefits from exercise when you work out in a fasted state—as such, an early morning burst of activity, pre break-fast, is ideal. Just how much your energy systems benefit from exercising on an empty stomach depends on your level of fitness (the less fit you are, the greater the potential benefit), but no matter your fitness level, exercising in a fasted state will help increase mitogenesis, reduce ROS production, and improve insulin sensitivity.[13] It doesn't hurt that exercise may also help to reduce appetite by changing the level of hormones that signal our sense of hunger.[14] I also think that pangs of hunger can partly be brought on by boredom, a feeling blunted by exercise.[15] So not only is this a good thing to do for your mitochondria, but as you start to implement your new chrono consumption schedule, you may find that exercising first thing in the morning helps you push back your eating window more comfortably. And starting the day with a quick workout is a surefire way to get your energy production in gear for the day ahead!

If you are new to exercise, you don't need to have any special equipment to start boosting your energy immediately. Simply move. Go outside and weed the garden or mow the lawn. Tidy up around the house. Jog in place for five minutes, or do jumping jacks. Use the back of a chair for balance and practice squats or lunges. Pick up a mini-trampoline (or rebounder—you can get one for under $30 these days) and jump on it for ten minutes. Rebounding is a wonderful low-impact activity that's easy on the joints and helps promote immunity and lymphatic drainage (toxin removal). There are all sorts of ways you can sneak a little more movement into your day—and the sum total of all of these exercise snacks can add up to big improvements.

If you're someone who likes to have a more specific program to start out, I've put together a little "snack circuit" for you below. Start off by completing this circuit twice a day or whenever you feel the need to get up and move your body, especially if you spend a large portion of your day sitting.

Exercise Snack Circuit

1. Jog in place. Just do a nice, easy trot for 1 minute. If this is too much for you, try it seated and move your legs and arms as though you're running.

2. Crunches. To do a crunch, lie on your back with your knees bent, and with either arms behind your head or arms pointed toward your feet, lift your head and shoulders up off the floor, then slowly lift your torso up, vertebra by vertebra. Go as far as you can go and do as many as you can within 1 minute without going too quickly; you want to keep your form the whole time, making sure your abs are doing the work, not your arms or neck.

3. Planks. Planks are a great all-around body strengthener, and they can be done practically anywhere. To do a plank, get into push-up position on the floor with arms and legs out straight, resting on your toes (or bended knees if you need the support). With your back straight, head and neck in a neutral position, and your hands directly below your shoulders, squeeze your glutes, abs, and quads for 1 minute. If you are new to the exercise, you may find it a bit challenging—take a break whenever you need to. A slightly modified version is to rest on your elbows with your forearms out front. Whichever position you choose, you should feel your core engaged. If planks aren't your thing, do a regular old or modified (knees on the floor) push-up.

4. Squats. This is another great move you can do anywhere. Stand with your feet parallel and a little wider than hip-width apart. Raise your arms to shoulder level, and as you squeeze in your abdominal muscles, slowly bend your knees while keeping your chest forward and your head lifted. Bend as deeply as your mobility will allow, then return to a standing position by engaging your gluteal muscles. Do as many repetitions as you can in 1 minute, focusing on keeping your form. Hold on to a counter or the back of a chair with one hand if you need balance.

From Snacks to Full Meals

If you're beginning from an advanced level of fitness or you're ready to move to the next level after practicing regular movement and exercise "snacks," you will certainly benefit from challenging your body even more. Longer cardio workouts as well as high-intensity interval training (HIIT) are two ways to increase your exercise from a snack to a full meal. Longer duration and higher intensity exercise are not essential components of the Energy Paradox

Program, but the more you can challenge your body, the more energy you will have.

HIIT is often described as an alternating series of short spurts of intense anaerobic exercise with brief recovery periods. There are many variations on the theme, but it can be as simple as doing some intervals on a stationary bike, running, or using a rowing machine. Here's how it works: You pedal, run, or row as fast as you can for 45 seconds, back off for 2 minutes, and repeat the circuit for as long as you can go. I personally do a HIIT bike training session at least once a week for 30 minutes. You can find multiple HIIT workouts offered on Instagram, YouTube, and any number of fitness apps, and there are many variations on the concept, so feel free to look around and see what appeals to you.

In addition to exercising with equipment like stationary bikes and rowing machines, I encourage you to take your training outside whenever possible. Because the more you expose your skin—and your eyes—to full-spectrum natural daylight, the more your mitochondria will benefit, and you'll sleep better too. Plus, who doesn't want to breathe in fresh air and feel the sun on their face when you're working up a sweat? It just feels good to move your body outside. Now let's take a look at some of the other benefits of spending time in the great outdoors.

Sunlight: Nature's Free Vitamin

I often tell my patients that they should think of sunlight as one of the most inexpensive and effective supplements out there. Exposure to sunlight helps your body produce vitamin D, which, as discussed in Chapter 3, is intimately connected with energy levels because it supports the intestinal wall integrity and immune function.[16] In addition, studies show there is a skin-gut axis at work here, with UVB rays from natural light offering benefits to the microbiome.[17] I also prescribe the sun for yet another reason: Full-spectrum natural light plays a critical role in our energy stores by giving our skin's melanin the power it needs to help make ATP (remember, we are more like plants than we think!). And with the help of the sun's infrared light, we can lower blood pressure while increasing overall blood flow.[18] As you likely have experienced, getting plenty of bright daylight also improves your mood and helps you sleep better at night. So get out there—the more you get those rays (yes, you get them even if it's overcast), the better your inner energy systems function.

I recommend exposing your skin to the sun for an hour a day, every day. In an ideal world, you want to bare as much skin as possible (I know, I know, easy to say if you're a guy who lives in Southern California!). Seriously, though, while I know that taking a stroll in a T-shirt and shorts may be a tough proposition in January, cold exposure is another beneficial stressor that activates hormesis—two birds, one stone!

Regular sun exposure is key not only to reaping the energy-boosting benefits of sunlight, but some suggest it may also (paradoxically?) be critical to protecting yourself from sun damage. In fact, Matt Maruca, a researcher in the field of photobiology and founder of blue-blocking eyewear brand Ra Optics, has spoken about emerging science on building up a "sun callus." Just like a callus you can get by learning to play guitar or walking barefoot—a protective buildup created by doing one thing over and over—Maruca cites how regular, moderate exposure to sunlight all year round has a protective benefit.[19] When we don't get adequate exposure to sunlight throughout the seasons, we step outside totally unprepared in the summertime and fry our cells, which can create carcinogenic damage and stress. Regular exposure to sunlight helps us build up a healthy callus, limiting the potential for skin damage while we safely benefit from the sun's multivitamin effects.

Eat Your Sunscreen

Your dermatologist has probably lectured you about applying sunscreen before you go outside for any amount of time, and the hazards posed by the UV rays are very real. That said, sunscreen completely blocks the sun's energy-producing rays, so if you wear sunscreen all the time, you simply cannot reap the sun's energy-giving benefits. (And if you're using conventional sunscreen that contains endocrine-disrupting chemicals, you're actually hurting your energy production! See page 156 for more information on safe sunscreen options.) Depending on where you live and your particular skin type, you may not need to use much sunscreen at all if you follow common-sense protocols.

You can also eat your sunscreen, like I do, to confer extra protection as you gradually build up that solar callus. No, I don't mean you should gulp down a bottle of SPF; rather, several naturally occurring compounds in a variety of foods offer protective properties from the sun (these compounds can also be taken in supplement form). Here are a few examples:

- **Lycopene**: This compound is commonly found in tomatoes, but you know how I feel about those lectin-rich nightshades! Cabbage, asparagus, and pink grapefruit (in season) are also rich in lycopene.
- **Omega-3 fatty acids**: To protect your skin from sun damage, eat omega-3 eggs, walnuts, wild salmon, flaxseeds, and purslane; better yet, take fish- or algae-based DHA, DPA, and EPA supplements.
- **Sulforaphane**: This compound found in cruciferous vegetables such as broccoli and arugula has been shown to reduce inflammation caused by UV radiation.[20]
- **Vitamin C**: I call vitamin C the "beauty nutrient" because there is very good evidence that vitamin C can prevent solar damage to the

skin.[21] Broccoli, kale, and other cruciferous veggies and lemon juice and zest are all packed with vitamin C. (Yes, lemon is a fruit, but it contains hardly any sugar.) To ensure you get enough vitamin C, I recommend taking a time-released supplement of 1000 mg twice a day.

Shutdown Mode: Turn off the Blue Light

We're not done with the sun just yet. As you may remember from Chapter 6, the sun regulates sleep and wake cycles, as well as our eating cycles. Before electricity, our ancestors ate according to daily and seasonal changes in sunlight exposure, not dissimilar to how the long days of blue light in the summer prompt bears to fill their bellies with berries and salmon, which will turn into fat that nourishes them through their long, sleepy winter. Like those bears, we are encouraged by warm, long days to increase our food consumption (including the only sweet food that was once available to us, fruit) so that we have extra fuel to burn during the leaner months. And while humans don't hibernate, traditionally the colder, shorter days and longer nights of winter meant fewer food options, less time for activities like hunting or gathering, and more time for rest and sedentary activity.

We existed this way for millennia. But the discovery of electricity and subsequent invention of artificial lighting profoundly disrupted these natural rhythms. Soon a variety of light-emitting devices—including televisions, computers, and eventually smartphones—came into existence. All of these gadgets are illuminated by *artificial* blue light, which in recent years has come to be referred to as "junk light." Blue light disrupts our circadian clock, and today it is hard to get away from. We stare into the blue lights of our devices long after sunset, while sitting in neighborhoods and cities that are illuminated by artificial light. Such environmental "light pollution" not only makes it hard to see the stars, it also interferes with melatonin regulation and makes it hard for us to fall asleep, because it sends our brain the message that it's time to be awake.

Another consequence of all this junk light exposure is weight gain. When our retinal cells detect blue light, they convey information to areas of the brain that regulate appetite and signal that it's time to eat (remember, historically we ate more in the summer and fall, when longer days meant more blue light). In one 2019 study, researchers exposed rats to nighttime blue light and then measured the rats' food consumption and glucose tolerance.[22] In order to better model human light exposure, the rats, which are typically nighttime feeders, were bred to be diurnal, meaning awake during the day and asleep at night, like humans. After only *one hour* of nocturnal blue light exposure, glucose tolerance was altered in male rats, a warning sign of prediabetes. In addition, when offered various food options, the rats chose to consume more sugary foods after exposure to the blue light. Hmm . . . is it a coincidence that you tend to reach for sweet snacks when you're binge-watching your favorite show? I don't think so. It would seem that junk light makes us reach for junk food.

In order to regain our energy—and our overall well-being—it is essential for us to reestablish our circadian rhythm and get back in sync with the natural ebb and flow of daylight. This means we must reduce our exposure to blue light as much as possible, and aim to expose our eyes to its natural counterbalance, *red* light, at sunrise and sunset. (Remember, the red and infrared wavelengths of the spectrum help your mitochondria do their work.) To mimic this, you can buy a red light device such as Joovv, which I personally use. You can also construct a simple light box with infrared light bulbs available at any hardware store. (On my website, you will find a podcast with the Joovv founders, who provide a lot of great information about ways to get more red light exposure.)

I realize that shutting off blue light in the evenings may not seem practical or enjoyable—it might be the only time of day you have to catch up on social media, or email, or just kick back and watch TV. Luckily, as fast as technology is moving, features that allow us to use our devices safely are keeping up pace. For instance, you can now download apps for just about any device that allow you to switch over to non–blue light at sundown and sunset (one of the best is from iristech.co), or if you have an iPhone you can switch it to "nighttime mode." If you're going to watch TV after dark—and I know you will—do yourself a favor and invest in a pair of amber-tinted blue blocker glasses that filter out the blue light (Ra Optics or BLUblox are two brands you could try). For best results, wear them from sundown until you go to sleep. You can also purchase special light bulbs you can use indoors and outdoors of your home that emit blue-depleted light (Lighting Science is a good, affordable brand).

And I hope it goes without saying that when you actually get into bed for some shut-eye, you must shut off your electronic devices—do not take them to bed with you! Some may emit blue light even when dormant, and they may also emit EMFs that disrupt sleep patterns, so plug them in to recharge on the other side of the room (better yet, outside of the room so you're not tempted to check Twitter during the middle of the night). And this brings us to the next "S" in our lifestyle plan, which is something many of my patients get too little of: sleep.

Sleep: Recharging Our Cells

Sleep (or the lack thereof) is a perfect example of "been down so long it looks like up to me." We are a nation of people walking around as sleep-deprived zombies, and we've become sadly accustomed to it. For many people, the shoe doesn't drop until true sleep deprivation starts to hit—by then, the damage has been accumulating for some time. As my good friend Arianna Huffington shared in her book *The Sleep Revolution*, she learned about the importance of sleep the hard way while trying to power through her days as the ultimate "super woman." After her chronic sleep-deprivation was to blame for a scary accident, she woke up.

The importance of good-quality and sufficient sleep cannot be underestimated; it is as critical to our well-being as nutrition, yet it is often—to use a wheel analogy—the one spoke that is broken. It is only recently that the scientific community has begun to fully appreciate the myriad ways sleep impacts our health, and my hope is that in sharing these benefits with the public, people start to prioritize their nightly shut-eye.

As you know, one obstacle to restful sleep is blue light, which affects your circadian clock and disrupts sleep patterns. In order to get the sleep your body needs, it's important to reestablish your circadian rhythm and get back in sync with the natural ebb and flow of daylight. But light isn't the only factor that gets in the way of a good night's sleep. In fact, the number one suggestion I give my patients who have trouble sleeping is to not eat within three hours of bedtime. As we discussed in Chapter 5, during sleep, your body engages in repair mode, and your brain in particular "cleanses" itself, a function that is essential to healthy cognitive and neurological function.[23] But the process of digestion diverts blood flow down to the gut instead of giving your brain the resources it needs for its freshening-up period. So, please, finish eating three hours before bedtime at least once a week, but ideally every day. You will be shocked how much better and deeper you will sleep.[24]

If you're someone who struggles with falling or staying asleep and you don't have a regular exercise habit, I also recommend you move your body more during the day. Sleep and exercise is a two-way street. Lack of sleep prevents you from exercising and vice versa—or to put it another way, few things help you sleep well like muscles that are tired from exertion.

Shut-eye Supplements

There's no harm in getting a little help to ease you into dreamland. But please be aware that not all sleep aids are alike—you want to take supplements that naturally gently help you nod off, not medications that alter your natural sleep cycle. Here are a few safe sleep aids I recommend to my insomniac patients:

Melatonin: This synthetic version of the hormone your body naturally produces at nighttime has long been known as a beneficial sleep supplement with few side effects. I don't necessarily recommend taking it every night as a crutch—you should be making the lifestyle changes described in this chapter, instead—but if your internal clock has been thrown off by travel or a hectic work schedule, I recommend taking time-released melatonin to help reset your natural sleep-wake cycle. The pills usually come in 3- to 5-mg doses—and that's plenty.

Relora: This blend of magnolia bark extract and *Phellodendron* (bark from a cork tree) also has remarkable sleep-restoring properties, while not being a sedative. If you happen to be one of the very few people who actually do have elevated cortisol levels, this supplement will help return your cortisol levels to normal. Take 300 mg two to three times per day.

Glycine: Glycine packs a one-two punch. It lowers body temperature when taken near bedtime (and a low body temperature is critical to induce sleep), and offers the added benefit of competing with glyphosate for binding sites in tissues. So while it helps you fall asleep, it is also working to protect you from any pesticide residue in your dinner! Take 1000 mg a day before bed.

Probiotics and prebiotics: I always keep some probiotics and prebiotics on hand when I'm traveling. Sometimes, just giving your gut bugs a boost can help reset your clock, especially when arriving in different time zones.

GABA, L-theanine, ashwagandha, valerian extract, and rosemary extract: If you have trouble sleeping, these supplements are all great add-ons to your nighttime routine. There are common sleep aids that blend all of these in one pill. Doses vary.

A little self-discipline can go a long way too, and I encourage people to be consistent with their sleep patterns. Suppress the urge for a binge-watching marathon and go to bed at the same time each night, or at least as often as possible. Make sure you get a full seven to eight hours of sleep. Remember, this is not a luxury; your brain, your body, and your gut buddies all depend on it. Stay on schedule, even on weekends. Sleeping in doesn't make up for time lost during the week; in fact, it actually throws off your entire circadian rhythm.

Sensory Challenges:
When Too Much of a Hard Thing Is a Good Thing

You know that you can activate hormesis through time-restricted eating and exercise, but as I hinted at earlier when I suggested you throw on some shorts and take a walk in the January sun, extreme sensory conditions—both cold and hot—are another way to induce your body's beneficial stress response. Research shows that such exposure makes our energy systems more efficient: As if in a nod to Darwin, our cells get the message that they had better toughen up if they want to survive, so they develop proteins as a means of protection. These proteins tell any cells that are not carrying their weight to self-destruct and recycle themselves (autophagy), leaving only healthy, fresh cells once the tide has turned and all is well again.[25] In addition, the shock to our system from extreme temperatures activates anti-inflammatory properties and increases production of our feel-good hormone, serotonin.

You may have heard of *cold therapy* or cryotherapy—a modality in which you strip down and step into a tank filled with subzero air, typically for a duration of two to four minutes. Cryotherapy offers many benefits, but it can be expensive and is not for everyone (if you do decide to try it, please do your research and find a certified practitioner!). You can achieve similar results by taking what is called a "scotch shower," where you crank up the cold water at the end of your shower for as long as you can take it (I suggest starting small and building up resilience). Now, a word of caution here. This is not for the "faint of heart"—POTS patients, or people with any heart condition (such as coronary artery disease, stents, pacemakers, or atrial fibrillation) should not try this, as it may cause cardiac arrhythmias and sudden dramatic dips of blood pressure.

You have greater stamina for the cold than you think—enduring it is just a matter of shifting your mindset, and exposing yourself to colder conditions regularly will help you build a greater tolerance. One way to get through the discomfort is to engage in breath work. In fact, an intensive breathing technique popularized by athlete Wim Hof has shown remarkable effectiveness in building tolerance to extreme cold. You can find free videos online that can help you learn this surprisingly easy and effective practice.

Some Like It Hot

Okay, so maybe you're more of a summer person. One great way to turn up the heat is to spend some time in a sauna. If you've experienced a good sauna session, you know it's a wonderfully relaxing (if sweaty) way to loosen up your muscles. Saunas are widely available and may even be free to use at your local health club, so they're a great, affordable option for temperature-induced hormesis. But if you're not a fan of the sweaty part (or sitting around half naked with a bunch of strangers), you can get a similar effect—and even more benefits for your mitochondria—from an infrared sauna.

Infrared saunas use electromagnetic infrared radiation to heat up the body's core temperature—in other words, the body heats up but not the air around it, and the temperature range is much milder. Infrared heating temperatures generally range from 110 to 120°F, compared to 160°F (or even higher) in a traditional sauna. And, without all that steam and humidity, they're a "dry" sauna. Infrared therapy is considered extremely safe—it's been used in hospitals for some time, even to warm newborn babies.

In addition to inducing hormesis, infrared saunas have been shown to have other energy-boosting effects, including helping to alleviate fatigue symptoms, most likely because of their ability to support normal blood pressure and circulation.[26] In fact, infrared saunas may give cardiovascular systems the same boost as exercising. The body starts sweating and your blood vessels dilate to increase blood flow. In one study of patients suffering from chronic fatigue syndrome, symptoms were dramatically improved after fifteen to twenty-five sessions of thermal therapy.[27]

So once a week or so, try to spend some time in a sauna or a steam room, expose yourself to a near-infrared or red-light sauna, take a hot yoga class, or come visit me in Palm Springs in the summer! If these options aren't realistic, simply take a nice hot bath. Recent studies have shown that a hot bath relieves mild depression better than antidepressants.[28] To avoid overstressing your cells, get into the bathtub when it's fairly warm, and then keep letting out some of the water and adding more hot water. You'll achieve the same hormetic effects as long as you're sweating.

Stress Management: Chill Out to Power Up

Historically, stress invaded our lives only in short bursts, and we had ample time for rest and recovery. Of course, the way stress affects our lives today is a different story altogether—stress is often chronic and unrelenting, and worse, we've normalized this state (much like being tired all the time) as the cost of modern life.

We know that the constant barrage of stress hormones in our body increases systemic inflammation, wreaks havoc on the gut, and is a major cause of brain inflammation (and resulting cognitive impairment) as well. Living with high levels of stress is simply not an option if we're going to reclaim our energy (and sanity). I realize this is easier said than done, but I want you to understand that stress is a very real physiological phenomenon with dangerous side effects.

So, let's talk about how you can manage your responses to today's seemingly endless stream of challenges. I always tell someone who's living with a lot of stress to start with two nonnegotiables:

daily exercise, which we know to be a powerful stress reducer, and fixing sleep deprivation. Once those habits are engrained, start bringing awareness to your stress response as it happens during the day. You have a lot more power over this than you realize! Your *conscious* thoughts can either activate your stress hormone network and, by association, your gut, or calm it all down. The easiest and cheapest way to calm your body's stress response is through controlled breathing. When you learn to "harness your breath" through conscious breathing, you tap into the power of your vagus nerve to calm your nervous system and communicate to your gut, and to your gut buddies, that "all is well." Breathing techniques are a free, easy, and remarkably effective way to manage stress.

My Favorite Breath Exercise

I mastered one of the simplest stress-busting tools in existence in my years as a surgeon. (Excuse the pun, but infant heart surgery is not for the faint of heart.) For the most part, I am focused and "in the zone" in the operating room, much like an athlete taking the field for a competition. But when something unexpected happens, I use controlled breathing to keep my heart rate steady and nervous system regulated. It looks like this:

Breathe in through your nose for a count of 3, then out through your mouth with pursed lips (like blowing out a candle) for a count of 6, repeating until you feel your tight breath deepen, your heart rate calm, and your mind more in control. In for 3, out for 6, in for 3, out for 6. Try it the next time you feel panic rising and I guarantee you will notice a difference!

In addition to breath work, I also recommend setting aside some time each day—maybe first thing in the morning, or last thing at night—to focus on the positive things in your life. I've spoken with a number of wonderful guests on my podcasts about this topic—a surprising number of very successful folks have mentioned that having a gratitude practice helps them manage their stress. Taking just a few moments to count your blessings has a remarkable effect, making it easier to get a handle on runaway negativity or ruminations. As challenging as it may be to recognize in a moment of struggle, there is always something to be thankful for.

In addition to focusing on gratitude, I would encourage anyone to experiment with meditation. There is very compelling evidence linking meditation to improved gut health—for one thing, it has been established that meditators have a far more diverse microbiome than people who don't meditate. And, the more diverse your microbiome, the better you can handle stress.[29] Meditation also offers deep moments of rest in short, concentrated bursts—for those who practice it, it's an energy lifesaver! These days, effective meditation practices are literally within arm's reach—there's a plethora of terrific apps available that can help you calm your mind.

But after you use your phone for a guided meditation, please put it down. Spend time away from social media and give yourself the gift of real-life social connection with those who are positive forces in your life. Sometimes nothing dispels stress better than an hour catch-up with a best friend or close sibling. We saw how Zoom calls between families and loved ones sustained people during the isolating experience of the pandemic—that innate need for connection truly helps our mood, which in turn helps everything in our body relax.

CHAPTER 9

ENERGY PARADOX RECIPES

Well, you've made it to the end, and I'll bet you're darn hungry by now. Luckily for you, I have a fresh batch of recipes to help you put the Energy Paradox Program into practice. These were developed with your mitochondria and your microbiome in mind. Remember, you are eating for them, not you, and that means plenty of prebiotic-, probiotic-, and postbiotic-producing foods that will keep them satisfied so they can help give you the energy you deserve. You'll notice a lot of shellfish, mollusk, and bivalve recipes, which will load you up with phospholipids, those backbones of your mitochondrial membranes. Hey, you're even going to try a shrimp cake for breakfast!

If you're a longtime Paradox devotee, keep in mind that all the recipes in my other books are Energy Paradox–compliant; just don't forget about the C^2 (chrono consumption) part of the energy equation, and modify any recipe that will serve as the first meal of the day so that it fits the description of a mono meal. To help you get started, I've put together a sample five-day meal plan to help you envision what your first week on the Energy Paradox Program might look like.

Sample Meal Plan

Day 1

Break-fast

A bowl of millet cereal with unsweetened almond milk

Lunch

Mushroom Soup 2.0 (page 243)

Dinner

Kate's Thanksgiving Salad (page 240)

Day 2

Break-fast

Fonio (millet), sorghum, or millet "oatmeal" made with unsweetened almond milk

Lunch

Kale, Broccoli, and Millet Burger with Creamy Avocado Sauce (page 252)

Dinner

Lectin-Free Fried Oysters and "Banh Mi" Bowl (page 255)

Day 3

Break-fast

4 egg whites, scrambled (feel free to add herbs of choice)

Lunch

Ground "Beef" Tacos (page 256)

Dinner

Spanish-Style Shellfish Stew (page 249)

Day 4

Break-fast

Hemp Green Protein Smoothie (page 239)

Lunch

Almost-Classic Clam Chowder (page 246)

Dinner

Mushroom and Shellfish Coconut Curry (page 248)

Day 5

Break-fast

Cauliflower Waffles (use the mono meal version, page 239)

Lunch

Instant Pot Lentil, Kale, Leek, and Mushroom Soup (page 245)

Dinner

Cauliflower Risotto with Scallops (page 247)

Snacks and Dessert

½ avocado with Miso-Sesame Dressing (page 261)

Small piece of in-season fruit

Mushroom Hot Chocolate (page 259)

Dark Chocolate Cauliflower Brownies (page 261)

Nuts

The Recipes

Break-fast

Lectin-free Cardamom Hazelnut Granola with Orange Zest

I've had quite a few patients struggle to give up their breakfast staple: yogurt with granola. So instead of forcing them to quit, I came up with a lectin-free, sugar-free alternative that's fantastic over unsweetened coconut yogurt. You can even sprinkle this granola over in-season fruit for a fruit crumble! Just keep in mind that this is not a mono meal, so please enjoy this after you've completed the first six weeks of the program.

Serves 8 to 10

2 cups roughly chopped hazelnuts

1 cup flaked unsweetened coconut

1/4 cup ground flaxseeds

1/4 cup sesame seeds

1/2 cup compliant butter (see page 200) or coconut oil

Zest of 2 oranges

1 teaspoon ground cardamom

1/4 teaspoon ground cinnamon

1/2 teaspoon salt

1/4 cup monkfruit sweetener

1/4 cup powdered Swerve sweetener

1/2 teaspoon vanilla extract

Preheat the oven to 300°F. Line a baking sheet with parchment or a silicone mat. Set aside.

In a large bowl, toss together the hazelnuts, coconut, flaxseeds, and sesame seeds. Set aside.

In a small saucepan, melt the butter. Add the orange zest, cardamom, cinnamon, salt, monkfruit, and Swerve and cook over low heat, stirring frequently, until the sweeteners are mostly dissolved. Remove from heat, then stir in the vanilla.

Pour the butter mixture over the nut mixture and stir until well combined.

Transfer the mixture to the prepared baking sheet and spread into a thin, even layer. Bake for 20 to 30 minutes, until golden brown and very fragrant, then remove from oven and let cool.

Break into bite-sized pieces, then store for 10 days at room temperature or 3 months in the freezer.

Sweet or Savory Cauliflower Waffles

Waffles made from cauliflower? It may sound unusual, but cauliflower makes a great base for just about any traditional carb-centric recipe, and now I've found a way to incorporate this gut-boosting cruciferous vegetable into waffles! Make sure to grease your waffle iron well, and handle these waffles with care—they tend to be a little fragile.

Serves 2

Waffle base:

3 cups cauliflower rice, finely pulsed in food processor

3 tablespoons almond flour

2 tablespoons coconut flour

3 large omega-3 eggs

Avocado oil spray

Fresh herbs or in-season fruit, for serving (optional)

For savory waffles, stir in:

1/4 cup Parmesan cheese

1 teaspoon paprika

1/2 teaspoon granulated garlic

3 tablespoons minced fresh chives

1 tablespoon minced fresh rosemary

For sweet waffles, stir in:

2 tablespoons almond flour

2 tablespoons coconut flour

1 1/2 teaspoons tapioca starch

2 tablespoons monkfruit or powdered Swerve sweetener

1 teaspoon ground cinnamon

Zest of 1 orange

In a large bowl, stir together the cauliflower rice, almond flour, coconut flour, and eggs from the base recipe.

Add the ingredients from either the sweet or savory variation (you must use one or the other) and stir to combine well.

Coat a waffle iron with avocado oil spray and heat over the medium heat setting. When the indicator light is on, spray again with the oil.

Pour 1 cup of the cauliflower mixture into the waffle iron, close, and cook for 5 to 7 minutes until deep golden brown.

Carefully remove the waffle, repeat with the remaining batter, and serve plain, with fresh herbs, or in-season fruit of choice.

Mono Meal Break-Fasts

Here are a few of my favorite ways to break the fast the mono meal way. Remember, whether you're eating protein, carbs, or (after week 2) fat for your first meal, you're easing your mitochondria into their workday so that they can produce energy for you as efficiently as possible.

Protein

Chicken Sausage Patties

Serves 2

Olive oil spray
1 shallot, minced
1 teaspoon poultry seasoning
1/4 teaspoon sweet paprika
1/2 teaspoon iodized sea salt
8 ounces ground pasture-raised chicken

Coat a large skillet with olive oil spray, then heat the skillet over medium heat.

Add the shallot, poultry seasoning, and paprika and mix until the mixture is fragrant and the shallot is tender. Transfer the mixture to a bowl and allow it to cool to room temperature. Wipe the pan clean and set aside (you'll use it again). Add the salt and chicken to the shallot mixture and mix to incorporate the seasonings into the chicken.

Shape mixture into 4 thin patties (like fast food–style burger patties) and set aside.

Spray the skillet with oil again and heat over medium-high heat. Add the patties to the pan and cook for 4 to 5 minutes per side (7 to 10 minutes if using dark meat), until an instant-read thermometer inserted into the center of each patty reaches 160°F. Remove from the pan and serve.

Shrimp Cakes

Serves 2 generously

14 ounces raw wild-caught shrimp, shells removed, finely chopped

2 ribs celery, diced

1/2 yellow onion, diced (save 1 teaspoon for the sauce)

2 cloves garlic, crushed

1 teaspoon Old Bay Seasoning

Zest of 1 lemon

2 tablespoons cassava flour, plus more if needed

1/4 cup omega-3 egg whites (2 eggs)

1/4 cup blanched almond flour

Avocado oil spray

In a large bowl, combine shrimp, celery, onion, garlic, Old Bay, lemon zest, cassava flour, and egg whites. The mixture should easily form cakes between your hands—if it falls apart, add more cassava, 1 teaspoon at a time, until it comes together.

Place the almond flour into a shallow bowl. Form the shrimp mixture into 4 equal-sized cakes, dip them into the almond flour, and gently pat to coat. Place on a plate and refrigerate for 15 to 20 minutes.

Coat a large skillet with avocado oil spray, then heat over medium-high heat. Cook the shrimp cakes until browned on the bottom, 3 to 4 minutes. Gently flip and cook for an additional 3 to 4 minutes to brown the other side. Reduce the heat to low and continue to cook until a sharp knife inserted into the center of a cake comes out hot, 1 to 2 minutes more.

Carbs

Millet and Strawberry Porridge

Serves 4 to 6

1¹/₂ cups uncooked millet

2 cups water

1 cup light unsweetened canned coconut milk

¹/₂ cup unsweetened, shredded coconut

¹/₄ cup monkfruit sweetener (optional)

1 teaspoon ground cinnamon

¹/₄ teaspoon ground allspice

¹/₂ teaspoon iodized sea salt

1 cup chopped organic strawberries (frozen are okay)

Zest of 1 lemon

Select the Sauté setting on your Instant Pot and let it heat up for a few minutes. Add the millet and toast, stirring frequently, until it smells nutty, about 5 to 6 minutes.

Add the water, coconut milk, shredded coconut, monkfruit, if using, cinnamon, allspice, salt, strawberries, and lemon zest and stir to combine. Lock the lid into place, select high pressure, and set the cook time to 10 minutes.

Select Cancel and allow the pressure to release manually. Open the lid, stir, and serve.

Cauliflower Waffles, Mono Style

Serves 2

3 cups cauliflower rice, finely pulsed in food processor

5 tablespoons almond flour

$1/4$ cup coconut flour

$1^1/_2$ teaspoons tapioca starch

2 tablespoons monkfruit sweetener

1 teaspoon ground cinnamon

Zest of 1 orange

6 egg whites (or 3 flax eggs)

Avocado oil spray

$1/_2$ cup fresh berries, for serving

In a large bowl, stir together cauliflower rice, almond flour, coconut flour, tapioca starch, monkfruit, cinnamon, and orange zest.

If using egg whites, in a small bowl, whip them until frothy. Combine the egg whites (or flax eggs) with the dry mixture and stir until a cohesive batter has formed. Let rest for 5 to 10 minutes for the coconut flour to hydrate.

Coat a waffle iron with avocado oil spray and heat over the medium heat setting. When the indicator light is on, spray again with the oil.

Pour 1 cup of the cauliflower mixture into the waffle iron (more for jumbo waffle irons), close, and cook for 5 to 7 minutes until golden brown.

Carefully remove the waffle, repeat with the remaining batter, and serve with berries on top.

Hemp Green Protein Smoothie

Serves 1

1 cup chopped romaine lettuce

$1/_2$ cup baby spinach

$1/4$ cup hemp hearts

1 mint sprig with stem

1/4 cup freshly squeezed lemon juice

3 to 6 drops stevia extract or 1 teaspoon allulose sweetener

1/4 cup ice cubes, plus more as needed

1 cup water

Combine all the ingredients in a high-powered blender and blend on high speed until smooth and fluffy, adding more ice cubes if you like.

Entrées

Kate's Thanksgiving Salad

People used to look at me funny when I suggested serving a salad at Thanksgiving—right until I served them this salad. It's one of those restaurant-style dishes that has so many "treats" hidden in it that every bite feels special and exciting.

Serves 4 generously

1 large sweet potato, peeled and cut into small cubes

2 cups sliced mushrooms (cremini or white button)

1/4 cup olive oil, divided

3 tablespoons minced fresh sage, divided

1 teaspoon iodized sea salt, plus more to taste

2 cups shredded Brussels sprouts (from about 6 ounces sprouts)

1 bunch of kale, stems removed, thinly sliced

2 cups broccoli slaw

1 bulb fennel, thinly sliced

Zest of 1 orange

Zest and juice of 1 lemon

2 shallots, minced

1 teaspoon ground black pepper

2 teaspoons Dijon mustard

3 tablespoons red wine vinegar

1/2 cup shredded Parmesan cheese (optional)

1 cup toasted hazelnuts

1/4 cup toasted sesame seeds

1 cup pomegranate arils (when in season)

Preheat the oven to 400°F.

In a large bowl, toss the sweet potato and mushrooms with 2 tablespoons of the oil. Add 1 tablespoon of the sage and a pinch of the salt.

Transfer the sweet potato mixture to a baking sheet and roast until the sweet potatoes are tender, 10 to 15 minutes. Remove from the oven and let cool to room temperature.

In a small saucepan, heat the remaining 2 tablespoons oil with the remaining 2 tablespoons sage over low heat. As soon as the sage smells fragrant, about 2 minutes, remove from the heat.

Meanwhile, toss the Brussels sprouts, kale, broccoli slaw, and fennel with the remaining salt. Rub the greens lightly between your hands to work in the salt. Let rest for 5 to 10 minutes.

Meanwhile, stir together the orange zest, lemon zest and juice, and shallots in a bowl. Add the black pepper, mustard, and vinegar to the shallot mixture and stir until the mustard is dissolved. Add the sage-infused oil and stir vigorously until dressing is emulsified.

Toss the dressing with the greens mixture, then add the sweet potatoes and mushrooms. Gently toss to combine, then top with the cheese, if using, hazelnuts, sesame seeds, and pomegranate arils and serve.

Mushroom Broth

With so many varieties of premade stock and broth available, it's easy to run to the store and buy whatever's on sale—but a lot of those broths are incredibly high in sodium and made with lectin-rich ingredients. Once you make this delicious mushroom broth, you'll fall in love—and never want to use anything else!

Makes about 2 quarts

1/4 cup avocado oil

4 shallots, roughly chopped

10 cloves garlic, roughly chopped

2 tablespoons fresh thyme leaves

Zest and juice of 1 lemon

1 pound fresh mushrooms (button, portobello, cremini, oyster, or a mix), diced

1/4 cup red or white miso

1/4 cup coconut aminos

8 ounces dried mushrooms (shiitake, trumpet, lobster, porcini, or a mix)

1 cup dry white wine*

1 tablespoon monkfruit sweetener

8 cups water

If you prefer not to use wine, add another cup of water to the mix instead.

In a large soup pot, heat the oil over medium-high heat.

Add the shallots, garlic, thyme, lemon zest and juice, and fresh mushrooms and cook, stirring frequently, until the mushrooms are well browned and fragrant. Add the miso, reduce the heat to medium-low, and cook, stirring frequently, until the miso mixture is well incorporated with the mushrooms. Add the coconut aminos, dried mushrooms, wine, and sweetener, then mix to combine.

Add the water, cover, and bring to a simmer. Lower the heat and simmer for 30 to 40 minutes, until the mushrooms are very tender and the broth has a well-developed mushroom taste.

Strain and use immediately, or cool, transfer to an airtight container, and refrigerate for up to 2 weeks or freeze for up to 3 months.

Garlicky Swiss Chard "Noodle" Soup

Garlic lovers, this is for you. The combination of sweet, nutty roasted garlic and sautéed garlic in this comforting soup is absolutely delicious. Pureed cauliflower creates a creamy base that pairs beautifully with the chard "noodles" for a hearty, satisfying wintery soup you'll want to keep on the menu all year long.

Serves 4

40 cloves garlic, peeled

1/4 cup extra virgin olive oil, divided

1 medium yellow onion, minced

2 ribs celery, minced

2 cups cauliflower florets

1 teaspoon fresh thyme leaves

1 teaspoon iodized sea salt, plus more to taste

1 teaspoon ground black pepper

6 cups Mushroom Broth (page 241)

1 cup unsweetened canned coconut cream

1/4 cup grated Parmesan cheese (optional)

2 cups thinly sliced Swiss chard leaves

Preheat the oven to 350°F.

Place 30 cloves of the garlic in a small baking dish and drizzle with 2 tablespoons of the oil. Cover with foil and roast for about 20 minutes, until the garlic turns a light golden brown.

Meanwhile, roughly chop the remaining 10 cloves of garlic.

Heat the remaining 2 tablespoons oil in a large soup pot over medium-high heat. Add the onion, celery, cauliflower, chopped garlic, thyme, salt, and pepper. Cook, stirring frequently, until the onion is wilted and mixture is fragrant, about 5 to 7 minutes.

Add the mushroom broth and bring to a simmer. Reduce the heat to low, cover, and simmer for 15 to 20 minutes, until the cauliflower is very tender.

Remove the pot from the heat and stir in the roasted garlic, coconut cream, and cheese, if using. Using an immersion blender, or working in batches in a standing blender, blend until smooth and creamy. Return the pot to the stovetop and turn the heat to low. Add the chard and stir until wilted.

Taste, adjust the seasoning or liquid as needed (depending on whether you like a thinner or thicker soup), and serve.

Mushroom Soup 2.0

I've had a variation on mushroom soup in almost all of my cookbooks—because I just can't get enough of it! If you want a more classic "cream of mushroom" you can skip the relish, but believe me, you'll be missing out. The relish can be made up to two days in advance.

Serves 8

For the soup:

1 large head cauliflower, outer leaves removed, coarsely chopped

1/4 cup extra virgin olive oil, divided

2 pounds mushrooms, finely diced

1 teaspoon fresh thyme leaves

1 teaspoon fresh rosemary leaves

Zest of 1 lemon

4 shallots, roughly chopped

2 cloves garlic, minced

2 ribs celery, diced

1¹/₂ teaspoons iodized sea salt

¹/₂ teaspoon ground black pepper

¹/₂ teaspoon onion powder

1 teaspoon Dijon mustard

1 tablespoon white miso paste

2 tablespoons tahini (sesame paste)

6 cups Mushroom Broth (page 241)

1 cup unsweetened canned coconut cream

For the relish:

1 cup sliced white button or cremini mushrooms

Zest of 1 orange

Zest and juice of 1 lemon

¹/₂ teaspoon iodized sea salt

¹/₄ cup minced fresh flat leaf or Italian parsley

1 clove garlic, minced

¹/₄ cup olive oil

Preheat the oven to 400°F.

In a large bowl, toss the cauliflower with 2 tablespoons of the oil.

Transfer the cauliflower to a baking sheet and roast for 15 to 20 minutes, until nutty and golden brown.

Meanwhile, heat the remaining 2 tablespoons oil in a large soup pot over medium heat. Add the mushrooms, thyme, rosemary, and lemon zest and cook, stirring frequently, until the mushrooms are browned at the edges and mixture is fragrant, 5 to 7 minutes.

Add the shallots, garlic, celery, salt, pepper, and onion powder and cook until the celery and shallots are tender, 2 to 3 minutes. Add the mustard, miso, and tahini and stir until well incorporated. Add the mushroom broth, bring to a simmer, then reduce the heat to low, cover, and simmer for 10 to 15 minutes, until mushrooms are tender.

While the soup is simmering, make the relish: Simply toss all ingredients in a large bowl and let sit at room temperature for 15 minutes to allow flavors to meld (or refrigerate for up to 2 days).

Transfer the roasted cauliflower to the soup mixture and blend (either in a standing blender or using an immersion blender) until smooth. Stir in the coconut cream and cook uncovered over medium-low heat until you've reached your desired consistency. Taste and adjust the seasonings to your liking. Serve the soup topped with the mushroom relish.

Instant Pot Lentil, Kale, Leek, and Mushroom Soup

This hearty vegan soup is zesty, fresh-tasting, and super-filling. It's even better the next day, after the flavors have had time to meld, but I suggest adding the mint and parsley right before serving to preserve their flavor. For some added decadence, top with a dollop of coconut cream.

Serves 6 to 8

1/4 cup extra virgin olive oil

1 large leek, cleaned and thinly sliced

2 shallots, minced

3 cloves garlic, minced

2 cups roughly chopped cremini or portobello mushrooms

1 teaspoon dried oregano

1 teaspoon iodized sea salt

1/2 teaspoon ground cumin

1/2 teaspoon ground cardamom

Zest of 1 lemon

Zest of 1 orange

2 tablespoons tomato paste (optional)

2 tablespoons tahini (sesame paste)

1 cup dried red lentils

8 cups Mushroom Broth (page 241) or vegetable broth

4 cups thinly sliced kale

1/4 cup fresh mint leaves, roughly chopped

1/4 cup fresh flat leaf or Italian parsley leaves, roughly chopped

Select the Sauté setting on your Instant Pot and let it heat up for a few minutes. Add the oil, leek, shallots, garlic, and mushrooms and cook, stirring frequently, until the mushrooms are tender, 3 to 5 minutes. Add the oregano, salt, cumin, and cardamom and cook until fragrant, 1 to 3 minutes. Add the lemon and orange zest and cook for an additional 1 minute, then stir in the tomato paste, if using, and tahini. Add the lentils and broth to the pot and stir well. Lock the lid into place, select high pressure, and set the cook time to 12 minutes.

Select Cancel and allow the pressure to release naturally for 10 minutes. Manually release the remaining pressure from the pot, then open the lid and add the kale. Reseal the pot and cook on high pressure for 2 minutes, then allow the pressure to release naturally for 5 minutes. Manually release the remaining pressure from the pot. Open the lid, stir in the mint and parsley, and serve.

Almost-Classic Clam Chowder

*I absolutely love a good, hearty clam chowder, but most are made with pota-
toes, milk, and other ingredients that are pretty unhealthy. Luckily, you can
still have an ultra-creamy, ultra-flavorful soup without the lectins.*

Serves 6 to 8

20 ounces canned clams

1/4 cup avocado oil

1 onion, finely minced

2 ribs celery, finely minced

1 cup finely diced celery root
  (celeriac)

3 cups cauliflower florets

1 teaspoon ground black pepper

1/2 teaspoon iodized sea salt, plus
  more to taste

1 cup bottled clam juice

1 teaspoon fish sauce

4 cups vegetable or chicken broth

2 cups full-fat unsweetened canned
  coconut milk

1 bay leaf

1 sprig thyme

Zest of 1 lemon

Minced fresh flat leaf parsley and
  chives, to garnish

Drain the clams, reserving the liquid, and roughly chop them. Refrigerate until ready to use.

In a large soup pot, heat the oil over medium heat. Add the onion, celery, celery root, and cauliflower and cook, stirring occasionally, until
the onion is tender and the vegetables are beginning to soften, 5 to 6
minutes. Add the pepper and salt and cook for 1 minute more. Add the
clam juice, reserved clam liquid, fish sauce, broth, and coconut milk to
the pot and bring to a simmer. Add the bay leaf, thyme, and lemon zest.
Reduce the heat to low and simmer for 20 to 30 minutes, until the mixture is fragrant and the cauliflower is extremely tender.

Remove from the heat and remove the bay leaf and thyme. Using an
immersion blender or in a standing blender, carefully blend the soup
halfway, until the broth is creamy but with some chunks remaining. Add
the clams and stir to combine. Cook over low heat until the clams are
warmed through. Serve the soup topped with minced herbs.

Cauliflower Risotto with Scallops

This dish is inspired by one of my favorite food memories—eating a rich, bright, lemony risotto in Italy with my absolute favorite person, my wife, Penny. I'm proud of how we captured the creaminess and texture of a classic risotto with cauliflower rice—and rounded out the dish with buttery scallops and asparagus for a filling, fresh-tasting meal.

Serves 4

1/4 cup avocado oil, divided

2 medium leeks, rinsed and thinly sliced

1/4 cup minced shallots

Iodized sea salt

1 (1-pound) package cauliflower rice

3 tablespoons arrowroot starch

2 cups Mushroom Broth (page 241)

1/2 cup coconut cream

Zest and juice of 2 lemons, divided

1/4 cup nutritional yeast or Parmesan cheese

1/4 cup minced fresh flat leaf parsley

1 pound wild-caught scallops, patted dry

8 ounces roughly chopped asparagus

Heat 2 tablespoons of the oil in a large saucepan over medium-high heat. Add the leeks and shallots and a small pinch of salt and cook until the leeks and shallots are translucent, 4 to 5 minutes. Add the cauliflower rice and cook for about 5 minutes, until cauliflower rice is tender and excess liquid has evaporated from pan, then add the arrowroot and stir for about 1 minute. Add the mushroom broth and bring to a boil; it should start to thicken fairly quickly (2 to 3 minutes).

Once the risotto is boiling and thickened, add the coconut cream and reduce the heat to maintain a bare simmer. Add half of the lemon zest and juice, the nutritional yeast (or cheese), and parsley and stir well. Set aside.

Wipe off the pan and fully dry, then heat the remaining oil over medium-high heat.

Pat the scallops dry with a paper towel, then season them with a pinch of salt. Transfer the scallops to the pan and sear until golden brown, 2 to 3 minutes per side. Remove from the pan and set aside.

Add the asparagus and remaining lemon zest and juice to the pan. Reduce heat to low and cook for 1 to 2 minutes, until the asparagus is vibrant green. Remove from the heat.

Serve the risotto topped with the scallops, asparagus, and any extra parsley.

Mushroom and Shellfish Coconut Curry

When I used to eat takeout more often, one of my go-tos was Thai food—I absolutely love a spicy red coconut curry. I suggest serving this flavorful curry over steamed cauliflower rice for a filling, satisfying meal. And if you're a vegetarian, skip the shellfish and swap in chopped hearts of palm—just add them to the pot with the kale.

Serves 8

1 tablespoon sesame oil (toasted or plain)

3 leeks, cleaned and finely chopped

2 cloves garlic, pressed or minced

1 tablespoon minced fresh ginger

2 cups sliced brown mushrooms

2 tablespoons Thai red curry paste

1 tablespoon tahini (sesame paste)

8 ounces mussels in the shell, beards removed

8 ounces clams in the shell (littleneck or cherrystone)

2 (14-ounce) cans unsweetened full-fat coconut milk

1/2 cup Mushroom Broth (page 241)

6 ounces wild-caught shrimp, peeled

1 1/2 cups packed thinly sliced kale

5 to 6 drops liquid stevia

1 tablespoon fish sauce or coconut aminos

Juice of 1 lime

1 small handful of fresh basil or cilantro leaves, chopped

Cauliflower rice, for serving (optional)

Heat the oil in a large soup pot over medium-high heat. Add the leeks and cook until tender and translucent, 3 to 5 minutes. Add the garlic and ginger and cook until translucent, about 2 to 3 minutes. Add the mushrooms and cook until tender, 4 to 6 minutes. Add the curry paste and tahini and stir until well incorporated. Cook for 1 to 2 minutes, until very fragrant. Add the mussels, clams, coconut milk, and mushroom broth and give it a stir. Cover and cook for 6 to 10 minutes, until the shells have opened.

Add the shrimp (or hearts of palm), kale, stevia, and fish sauce (or coconut aminos), cover, and cook for an additional 4 to 6 minutes, until the shrimp are cooked through and the kale is wilted. Uncover and simmer for 3 to 4 minutes, until thickened slightly. Add the lime juice and basil or cilantro and serve over cauliflower rice, if desired.

Spanish-Style Shellfish Stew

This delicious stew is inspired by zarzuela, *the classic dish from the Catalan region of Spain. In my opinion, the saffron really makes the dish (and a little goes a long way), but if you can't find it, or if it's out of budget, I suggest adding a small pinch of turmeric for color.*

Serves 4 to 6

1 pound medium shrimp with shells

1/2 cup dry white wine

Large pinch of saffron

1/4 cup extra virgin olive oil

1/4 cup diced prosciutto (optional)

1 large onion, diced

1 rib celery, diced

1 white sweet potato, peeled and diced

2 cups cauliflower florets

1/2 teaspoon ground black pepper

1/2 teaspoon smoked paprika

1/2 teaspoon iodized sea salt, plus more to taste

6 cloves garlic, minced

1 tablespoon minced fresh rosemary

1 tablespoon fresh thyme leaves

1/2 cup peeled, seeded tomato puree, such as Pomi (optional)

5 cups fish stock, Mushroom Broth (page 241), or vegetable stock

1 pound Manila clams, cleaned

1 pound mussels, cleaned and debearded

3 bay leaves

1/4 cup almond meal

Juice of 1 lemon

1/4 cup minced fresh flat leaf parsley

Peel the shrimp and place the shells in a small saucepan. Refrigerate the shrimp until ready to use.

Pour the wine over the shrimp shells and add the saffron to the pan. Bring to a simmer over low heat, cover, and simmer for 15 to 20 minutes, until the saffron has bloomed and the shrimp shell flavor has been extracted. Set aside.

Meanwhile, heat the oil in a large soup pot over medium heat. If using prosciutto, add to the pan and cook for 3 to 4 minutes, stirring frequently, until the fat has rendered and the meat has crisped. With a slotted spoon, remove the meat from the oil and reserve for later.

Add the onion and celery to the soup pot and cook, stirring frequently, until the onion is translucent, 2 to 3 minutes. Add the sweet potato, cauliflower, pepper, paprika, salt, garlic, rosemary, and thyme and cook, stirring frequently, until very fragrant, 2 to 3 minutes. Add bay leaves, and the tomatoes, if using, and cook for an additional 2 to 3 minutes. Add the broth to the pan, reduce the heat to low, and cook covered for 10 to 20 minutes, until the cauliflower and sweet potato are very tender.

Using a wire strainer, strain the wine mixture into the pot, discarding the shells, bay leaves, and saffron threads. Add the shrimp, clams, mussels, and almond meal and simmer for 7 to 10 minutes, until the shrimp is pink and cooked through and the shellfish has opened. Add the lemon juice and parsley and the reserved prosciutto, if using, and stir. Serve immediately.

Shockingly Healthy Broccoli Casserole

I grew up in the Midwest—land of the casserole. And if I'm being honest, a cheesy, crunchy-topped casserole is one of my favorite guilty pleasures. So I went ahead and converted the classic Midwest broccoli-cheddar casserole into something that's actually good for your body (and still pretty indulgent!).

Serves 6

Olive oil spray

2 cups macadamia nuts, soaked overnight in water to cover

8 cups broccoli florets

1/4 cup olive oil, divided

1 onion, minced

1 cup finely minced mushrooms

1 (14-ounce) can full-fat unsweetened coconut milk

1/2 cup Mushroom Broth (page 241)

Juice of 1/2 lemon

1/4 cup nutritional yeast

1 teaspoon Dijon mustard

1 teaspoon onion powder

1/2 teaspoon ground black pepper

11/2 teaspoons iodized sea salt, divided

11/2 teaspoons avocado oil

1 cup crushed sweet potato or cassava chips

1/2 cup finely chopped walnuts

1 teaspoon finely minced fresh rosemary

Preheat the oven to 425°F. Spray a 9 x 13-inch casserole dish with oil (or brush with olive oil) and set aside.

Strain the macadamia nuts and set aside.

In a large bowl, toss the broccoli with 2 tablespoons of the olive oil. Spread the broccoli on an unlined baking sheet and roast until tender and beginning to brown around the edges, 10 to 20 minutes.

Reduce the oven temperature to 350°F and remove the broccoli from the oven.

While the broccoli is roasting, heat the remaining 2 tablespoons of olive oil in a large sauté pan over medium-high heat. Add the onion and mushrooms and cook until the onion is tender and the mushrooms are golden brown.

Remove the onion mixture from the heat and toss with broccoli mixture. Transfer to the prepared baking dish. Wipe pan clean with a dry towel, and set aside.

Make the "cheese" sauce: In a food processor fitted with an "S" blade, pulse the strained macadamia nuts until finely ground. Add the coconut milk, mushroom broth, and lemon juice and process until smooth and creamy, 2 to 3 minutes. Add the nutritional yeast, mustard, onion powder, pepper, and half of the salt, and process until smooth and creamy (thin out with water or broth as needed until you reach a nacho cheese sauce consistency). Pour the "cheese" mixture over the broccoli, and toss to combine well. Set aside.

In the sauté pan, heat the avocado oil over medium heat. Add the chips, walnuts, rosemary, and the rest of the salt, and cook, stirring frequently, until the nuts are toasty and the rosemary is fragrant.

Top casserole with the nut mixture, transfer to the oven, and bake until bubbling, 25 to 30 minutes. Serve immediately.

Broccoli-Kale Pesto

One of the best ways to use leftover green vegetables is to whiz them into a pesto. I love the sweetness that broccoli adds to this sauce, and I find that it balances very well with slightly bitter kale and buttery sesame seeds. You can use this pesto in any number of ways. Try tossing it with Miracle Noodles or sweet potato noodles or serving it as a dip with raw vegetables.

Makes about 1 1/2 cups

1/2 cup lightly steamed broccoli florets, cooled

1/2 cup thinly sliced lacinato kale leaves

1/4 cup loosely packed fresh basil leaves

1/4 cup loosely packed fresh flat leaf parsley leaves

1 small clove garlic, peeled

1/4 cup toasted sesame seeds (or 2 tablespoons tahini)

1/4 cup Parmesan cheese or nutritional yeast

1/2 cup extra virgin olive oil

Iodized sea salt

In a food processor fitted with an "S" blade, pulse together the broccoli, kale, basil, parsley, and garlic until well combined. Add the sesame seeds (or tahini) and cheese (or nutritional yeast) and continue to pulse until just combined and the mixture is still a little chunky. With the food processor running, stream the oil into the broccoli mixture until combined. Taste and add salt as needed.

Kale, Broccoli, and Millet Burger with Creamy Avocado Sauce

I'm always on a mission to make the perfect veggie burger, and if you've tried the ones in my other cookbooks, you know: I've created some delicious ones. But the beautiful thing about veggie burgers is that they are endlessly adaptable. This broccoli-and-kale version will be a hit with all of you cruciferous vegetable lovers!

Note: Omit the sauce and this becomes a great break-fast mono meal.

Makes 4 patties

For the sauce:

2 ripe avocados, cut in half, pitted, flesh scooped out

Juice of 1 lemon

1 clove garlic, peeled

1/4 cup chopped fresh dill

1/4 cup chopped fresh parsley

1/2 teaspoon iodized sea salt

1 shallot, minced

2 tablespoons capers

For the patties:

1 tablespoon avocado oil, plus more for cooking

2 shallots, minced

1 rib celery, minced

1 tablespoon minced fresh rosemary

1 cup roughly chopped kale leaves

1 1/2 cups steamed broccoli, cooled

1/4 cup chopped fresh flat leaf parsley

1/2 teaspoon iodized sea salt

1/2 teaspoon paprika

1/2 teaspoon garlic powder

1 teaspoon Dijon mustard

1 tablespoon tahini (sesame paste)

1 cup cooked millet (a little overcooked is fine—leftovers work great for this)

1/2 cup millet flour, plus more as needed

First, make the sauce: In a food processor fitted with an "S" blade, combine the avocado, lemon juice, garlic, dill, parsley, and salt and process until smooth and creamy. Add water, a teaspoon at a time, to achieve a spreadable consistency if it doesn't come together on its own.

Fold in the shallot and capers. Cover and refrigerate until ready to use.

Preheat the oven to 375°F. Brush a baking sheet with oil or line it with parchment paper. Set aside.

Next, make the burger patties: Heat the oil in a large sauté pan over medium heat. Add the shallots, celery, and rosemary and cook until fragrant, 1 to 2 minutes. Add the kale and continue to cook until the kale is wilted and tender, 3 to 5 minutes.

Add the steamed broccoli to the pan, then add the parsley, salt, paprika, and garlic powder. Cook, stirring frequently, until fragrant and well combined, 1 to 2 minutes.

Transfer veggie mixture to a food processor fitted with an "S" blade and pulse until no large chunks remain (rice consistency or a little smaller). Add the mustard and tahini and pulse until just combined.

Transfer the mixture to a large bowl and add the millet. Fold it in until it comes together.

Add the flour, half at a time, until a bit of the mixture squeezed in your hand forms a cohesive ball that's easy to shape (you'll likely need most of the flour).

Measure 1/2-cup portions of veggie mixture and shape it into patties. Place them on the prepared baking sheet and brush the tops of the burgers with oil. Bake for 12 to 15 minutes, until the tops are beginning to brown. Carefully flip the burgers and bake for an additional 10 minutes, until golden brown and crisp at edges.

Serve with avocado sauce, in a lettuce wrap, or as is.

Almond and Herb–Baked Mussels

These mussels are perfect for your next dinner party—they're a great one-handed appetizer, they're easy to make, and they feel fancy. I prefer to use fresh mussels, but I've also made these with frozen ones from Costco.

Serves 2 to 4 as a main, 4 to 6 as a side/appetizer

Avocado or olive oil spray

2 pounds mussels, well-scrubbed, beards removed

1 cup water

1 tablespoon extra virgin olive oil

6 cloves garlic, minced

1 tablespoon finely minced fresh rosemary

3/4 cup finely chopped blanched almonds

1/4 cup minced fresh flat leaf or curly parsley

1/4 cup Parmesan cheese or nutritional yeast

1/2 teaspoon paprika

Preheat the oven to 400°F. Spray a baking sheet with oil and set aside.

Place the mussels in a large skillet with a tight-fitting lid and add the water.

Cover and steam over medium heat, shaking the pan occasionally, until the mussels open—as long as 15 minutes, or as little as 5 minutes. As the mussels open, remove them from the pot and transfer them to a clean plate. Discard any mussels that haven't opened (it happens).

While the mussels cool, heat the oil in a medium sauté pan over medium heat. Add the garlic and rosemary and cook, stirring frequently, until the garlic is nicely toasted, about 2 to 3 minutes. Add the almonds and continue to cook until the almonds are toasty and browned, about 1 to 2 minutes. Remove from the heat and let cool.

While almond mixture is cooling, remove the top shells from each mussel and arrange each mussel open-side up on the prepared baking sheet. If you have trouble keeping them upright, try using foil to hold them in place (or spread the whole sheet with a layer of salt and nestle the shells in the salt).

Fold the parsley, cheese (or nutritional yeast), and paprika into the almond mixture. Carefully spoon the "crumb" mixture into each mussel, covering the meat completely.

Spray the mussels with oil and bake for 10 minutes, or until very golden brown. Remove from the oven and serve.

Lectin-Free Fried Oysters and "Banh Mi" Bowl

There's nothing like a crispy fried oyster—especially when served with an herbal, tangy, banh mi–inspired salad. Unfortunately, there's not a great vegan alternative to the oysters, though you can prepare artichoke hearts in a similar manner and they're pretty delicious—just use a flax egg rather than the real thing (and substitute coconut aminos for the fish sauce in your "bahn mi").

Serves 2 to 4

For the oysters:

12 fresh-shucked oysters (about 8 ounces)

1/2 cup tapioca flour, divided

1/4 cup almond flour

1/4 cup Parmesan cheese or nutritional yeast

1 tablespoon Old Bay Seasoning

1 large omega-3 egg

1 teaspoon Dijon mustard

Avocado oil, for frying

Iodized sea salt

For the "banh mi" bowl:

Juice of 1 lime

2 tablespoons fish sauce

1 teaspoon monkfruit sweetener

1 clove garlic, minced

1 carrot, thinly sliced

1 shallot, thinly sliced

2 cups salad greens

$1/2$ avocado

$1/4$ cup roughly chopped fresh mint leaves

$1/4$ cup roughly chopped fresh basil leaves

Fried oysters (see above)

Your favorite hot sauce and/or freshly squeezed lime juice

To make the oysters: Place the oysters in a strainer to strain out extra liquid.

In a bowl, toss together $1/4$ cup of the tapioca flour, the almond flour, cheese (or nutritional yeast), and Old Bay until well combined.

In a separate bowl, whip together the egg and mustard until well combined and frothy.

Dip the drained oysters into the remaining $1/4$ cup tapioca flour, then into the egg mixture, then into the tapioca-almond mixture. Set on a wire rack or paper towel.

Fill a large pan with about 1 inch of oil and heat over medium-high heat until the oil begins to pop. Gently transfer the oysters into the pan and cook for 1 to 2 minutes per side, until the oysters are golden brown. Transfer to a paper towel to cool. Sprinkle with salt right before serving.

To make the "banh mi" bowl:

In a bowl, combine the lime juice, fish sauce, monkfruit, and garlic, stirring until the monkfruit dissolves. Add the carrot and shallot and let marinate for 15 to 20 minutes, until they pickle slightly.

When the veggies are pickled, toss the veggies and the marinade together with the salad greens. Top with the avocado, chopped herbs, and fried oysters. Drizzle with hot sauce and/or a squeeze of lime before serving.

Ground "Beef" Tacos

A vegan taco that doesn't rely on processed fake meat? Not only is it possible, but it's totally delicious. And thanks to the mix of hearty walnuts and mushrooms, it's incredibly filling too. I suggest serving these tacos in lettuce leaves, but if you want to indulge, check out Siete cassava tortillas.

Serves 4

For the "meat":

1 cup chopped walnuts

2 pounds mushrooms (cremini, portobello, or white button)

1/4 cup olive oil

1 red onion, minced

2 cloves garlic, minced

1 tablespoon ground cumin

1 1/2 teaspoons chili powder

1 teaspoon dried oregano

1 1/2 teaspoons fish sauce or coconut aminos

1 tablespoon tahini (sesame paste)

Iodized sea salt

For the slaw:

1/4 cup red wine vinegar

2 tablespoons monkfruit sweetener

1/2 teaspoon iodized sea salt

2 carrots, finely shredded

1 red onion, thinly sliced

2 cups finely shredded cabbage

1 tablespoon Dijon mustard

2 tablespoons tahini (sesame paste)

2 tablespoons avocado mayonnaise

For the salsa:

2 ripe avocados, cut in half, pit removed, flesh scooped out

Juice of 2 limes

Juice of 1 lemon

1/4 cup fresh flat leaf parsley or cilantro leaves, finely minced

1 clove garlic, crushed

1 shallot, finely chopped

1/2 teaspoon iodized sea salt

To serve:

12 butter lettuce leaves

1/4 cup shredded goat cheddar (optional)

1/4 cup unsweetened canned coconut cream (optional)

To make the "meat": Pulse the walnuts and mushrooms in a food processor (or chop very finely with a knife) until they're broken into small crumbly bits (like ground beef crumbles).

Heat the oil in a large sauté pan over medium heat. Add the onion and garlic and cook, stirring frequently, until the onion is translucent and the garlic is fragrant, 2 to 3 minutes.

Add the walnut mixture, then add the cumin, chili powder, and oregano and continue to cook until the mixture is very fragrant, the spices are well combined, and the mushrooms are tender, 6 to 10 minutes.

Add the fish sauce (or coconut aminos) and tahini and cook until well combined. Taste and add salt as needed. Cover, set aside, and prepare the additional elements for the dish (this "meat" is best slightly warmer than room temperature).

To make the slaw: Combine the vinegar, monkfruit, and salt in a small saucepan and heat until the sweetener and salt have dissolved and the vinegar is hot. Add the carrot and onion, turn off the heat, and cover. Set aside for 5 to 10 minutes to allow veggies to pickle slightly and the vinegar mixture to cool.

Remove the vegetables from the vinegar, reserving the vinegar. Toss pickled vegetables with the cabbage.

Whisk the mustard, tahini, and mayonnaise into the vinegar mixture to make a dressing. Pour the dressing over the slaw and toss to combine.

To make the salsa: In a food processor, combine the avocados, lime juice, and lemon juice and process until creamy and smooth. Add the parsley (or cilantro), garlic, shallot, and salt and pulse a couple times, until just combined but still chunky. Add water, as needed, to reach a thick but pourable salsa consistency. Chill until ready to serve (you'll only need half of the salsa for this recipe).

To assemble the tacos: Spoon the "meat" mixture into each lettuce leaf and top with the slaw and a drizzle of salsa. Add the cheese and coconut cream, if using. Feel free to invite everyone at the table to fix their tacos as they like.

Sweets and Snacks

Mushroom Hot Chocolate

Mushrooms in your cocoa?! I know, it sounds strange, but it's so good! This hot drink is a wonderful dessert alternative, delicious mixed in with coffee, or, if you use coconut milk, you can chill it for a rich chocolate pudding. What a great way to get your melatonin and polyamines!

Serves 2

2 tablespoons mushroom powder (chaga, reishi, cordyceps, or make your own*)

1/4 teaspoon ground cinnamon

1 star anise pod (optional)

1 scant pinch of iodized sea salt

1 ounce bittersweet chocolate (72% cacao or higher), diced

1 1/2 cups unsweetened coconut milk, almond milk, or hazelnut milk

*To make your own mushroom powder, place dried, dehydrated mushrooms in a blender, food processor, or spice grinder and pulse until finely powdered. Shiitake, porcini, trumpet, and oyster mushrooms are widely available and work well for this recipe.

In a small saucepan, whisk together the mushroom powder, cinnamon, star anise, if using, and salt. Add the chocolate and milk to the pan and cook over low heat, whisking constantly so the chocolate doesn't burn, 3 to 5 minutes.

When the mixture is hot and the chocolate is melted, strain through a fine-mesh strainer into the mug of your choice and enjoy.

Basil Seed Pudding

Chia seed pudding has been a food trend for a few years now, but, unfortunately, chia seeds are terrible for your gut. Enter the humble basil seed! Yep, the same one you use in your herb garden. Look for them in well-stocked Asian markets or online, where you may find them labeled as sabja, tukmaria, or falooda. I've included two different basil seed puddings, both of which are mono meals after week 2.

Coconut Lime Pudding

Serves 4

2 cups full-fat, unsweetened canned coconut milk

2 tablespoons monkfruit sweetener

Zest of 1 lime

$1/2$ teaspoon vanilla extract

$1/4$ teaspoon coconut extract

$1/4$ cup basil seeds

$1/4$ cup toasted coconut flakes

In a large saucepan, heat the coconut milk with the monkfruit over medium heat, stirring occasionally, until the monkfruit is dissolved. Reduce the heat to low, add the lime zest, stir, and cook until fragrant. Remove the mixture from the heat and add vanilla and coconut extracts and basil seeds. Stir the mixture, then let stand for 5 minutes for the seeds to absorb the liquid.

Stir well again, then transfer to 4 individual serving dishes and let set for at least 3 to 4 hours in the fridge. Top the pudding with coconut flakes before serving.

Chocolate Hazelnut Pudding

Serves 4

$1/2$ cup toasted hazelnuts, divided

2 cups full-fat, unsweetened canned coconut milk

2 ounces bittersweet chocolate (at least 72% cacao), diced

$1/2$ teaspoon vanilla extract

1 scant pinch of iodized sea salt

$1/4$ cup basil seeds

In a food processor or blender, process $1/4$ cup of the hazelnuts until a creamy hazelnut butter forms. Chop the remaining $1/4$ cup hazelnuts and set aside.

In a large saucepan, heat the coconut milk and chocolate over low heat, stirring occasionally, until the chocolate is dissolved. Remove the mixture from the heat and add the vanilla and salt. Add the basil seeds, stir, then let stand for 5 minutes for the seeds to absorb the liquid.

Stir well again, then transfer to 4 individual serving dishes and let set for at least 3 to 4 hours in the fridge. Top the pudding with reserved chopped hazelnuts before serving.

Raw Veggies with Miso-Sesame Dressing

This is my go-to dressing for any salad, and it also makes for a great dip for fresh veggies when you're craving a savory, umami-rich snack (you can add a little more miso paste to get a thicker consistency for dipping). The sweet-tangy taste is addictive!

Makes 1/2 cup

1/4 cup toasted sesame oil

2 tablespoons white miso paste

Juice of 1 lime

2 tablespoons rice wine vinegar

1 tablespoon coconut aminos

1 teaspoon grated fresh ginger (optional)

In a large bowl, whisk the oil and miso paste until smooth and creamy. Add the lime juice, vinegar, and coconut aminos and continue to whisk until well combined. Fold in the ginger, if using, then serve with fresh vegetables such as broccoli, cauliflower, endive, asparagus, and celery. The dressing can be stored in the fridge for up to 1 week. Whisk again before serving.

Dark Chocolate Cauliflower Brownies

This is one of those sneaky recipes that's great if you want to get your kids to eat their veggies. But even if you're an adult and you know perfectly well that there's cauliflower in these brownies, chances are, you won't be able to stop eating them!

Serves 12

1 cup cauliflower rice

1/2 cup full-fat unsweetened canned coconut milk

4 ounces 90% cacao chocolate, cut into chunks

1/3 cup coconut oil

2 tablespoons organic cream cheese, Italian mascarpone, or unsweetened coconut cream

2/3 cup monkfruit sweetener

2 omega-3 eggs or flax eggs

2 cups almond flour

1/4 teaspoon iodized sea salt

3/4 teaspoon baking powder

1/4 cup non-Dutched (natural) cocoa powder

1/2 cup chocolate chips (72% cacao or higher)

Preheat the oven to 350°F. Line an 8-inch square baking pan with parchment paper and set aside.

In a blender or a food processor fitted with an "S" blade, process the cauliflower rice and coconut milk until smooth and creamy; set aside.

Over a double boiler, or in a microwave in 10-second bursts, melt the chocolate together with the coconut oil, stirring frequently to prevent burning. When the chocolate is fully melted, remove from the heat and fold in the cauliflower mixture.

In a stand mixer, or using a large bowl and a whisk, beat together the cream cheese (or alternative) and monkfruit until fluffy and well combined. Add the eggs, one at a time, whipping to combine fully. Fold the cauliflower mixture into the egg mixture, whisking to combine.

In a separate bowl, whisk together the almond flour, salt, baking powder, and cocoa powder.

Add the dry ingredients to the wet ingredients and fold until well combined but not overmixed. Fold in the chocolate chips, then transfer to the prepared baking pan. Bake for 25 to 35 minutes, until a toothpick inserted into the center of the mix comes out with only a few crumbs stuck to it. Let cool completely (and preferably refrigerate) before slicing.

CHAPTER 10

THE ENERGY PARADOX
SUPPLEMENT LIST

Earlier in the book I warned about the overreliance on supplements to rid us of sluggishness, brain fog, and all-around fatigue. Some people, so desperate to feel better, will practically hand over their life savings to get their hands on the latest "wonder" supplements, that in the end probably won't help them. But I am in no way against supplements altogether, not by a long shot. I believe they can do a lot of good when they are used to *supplement* an underlying healthy diet and lifestyle that promotes energy.

The good news is that by following the program in this book, you will build a healthy foundation that allows a few simple supplements to do further work in helping lessen inflammation, maintaining a healthy microbiome, and maximizing ATP production. While I've included supplement recommendations in all of my Paradox books, the list that follows includes my essentials for boosting energy.

Magnesium

Many people are magnesium deficient, yet magnesium is critical to so many functions in the body—including strengthening metabolic health, improving sleep, and blocking the effects of EMFs. Magnesium can also help ease muscle cramps, which may occur as you begin the Energy Paradox Program. When you shift over to burning fat as a fuel, you will have used up glycogen in your muscles. Since glycogen is stored with water, magnesium, and potassium, when it is removed, out goes the magnesium and potassium with it!

Magnesium helps to bolster metabolic flexibility by helping insulin to get sugar out of your bloodstream and into your muscle cells, where it belongs, which in turn will help in reversing insulin resistance. I recommend potassium magnesium aspartate combinations, but if taking separately, I suggest 299 to 300 mg of magnesium and 99 mg of potassium twice a day. If magnesium gives you diarrhea, use an Epsom salt foot soak or bath or rub magnesium oil spray on your legs or belly.

Glycine

Glycine is an important amino acid supplement that can help protect us against the gut-harming effects of glyphosate (the dangerous ingredient in Roundup and other herbicides) and also has some antiaging properties.[1] Additionally, glycine helps to promote a better night's sleep; studies show that glycine ingestion before bedtime has been shown to significantly improve subjective sleep quality in individuals with insomniac tendencies, by causing a drop in body temperature. One study showed that rats who were given glycine experienced a significant decrease in core body temperature, which might help explain why it promotes better sleep. I recommend taking 1000 mg before bed as a sleep aid and/or 2000 mg a day as an antiaging anti-glyphosate aid.

Phospholipids

These complex fats are lipid molecules that compose much of our cellular and mitochondrial membranes. A recent study found that phospholipid supplementation may reduce fatigue in humans by as much as 40 percent(!).[2] These important phospholipids can be obtained in the diet from bivalves and shellfish or supplemented with krill oil. Look for a brand with the highest concentration of phospholipids per capsule. Choline, phosphatidylcholine, and phosphatidylserine are other phospholipids available in supplement form, in a dose of 500 to 1000 mg per day.

Vitamin K$_2$

An essential cofactor in mitochondria function, this vitamin is sadly missing from our modern diet. You can find it in grass-fed milk products, including butter and cheeses, but I recommend limiting dairy products and instead taking a K$_2$ supplement. A daily dosage of 100 mcg of both MK-4 and MK-7 varieties of vitamin K$_2$ should suffice.

Coenzyme Q10 (CoQ10), or Ubiquinol, or PQQ

These are all supplementary forms of an important coenzyme in the mitochondrial electron transport chain, which are essential for making energy! In general, 100 to 300 mg of CoQ10, 100 mg of ubiquinol, or 20 mg of PQQ is a good dose for mitochondrial support. If you are taking a statin drug, you are likely depleted in this coenzyme and need a higher dose; I recommend increasing levels of CoQ10 to 300 mg in this case.

Chlorella and Activated Charcoal

As was shown in the Biosphere 2 experiment, rapid weight loss (approximately a pound a week) releases heavy metals that cannot be properly detoxified by the liver and are instead excreted in bile and reabsorbed in our intestines, creating a vicious cycle; hence they must be bound up in our intestines to prevent reabsorption. In my clinics, I have achieved dramatic reductions in heavy metals like mercury, lead, and cadmium by using a combination of cracked cell chlorella (a great source of iodine as well) and activated charcoal, both of which help bind the toxic stuff for safe excretion. These are in my Untox formula, but can be found in most health food stores or online. Suggested doses are 500 to 3000 mg chlorella and 50 to 100 mg activated charcoal daily. A word of caution: I suggest limiting charcoal use to two months; take while you are on a fast and up to a month afterward. You do not want to stay on it too long, as it is such a good binding agent that it may start binding to the good stuff (vitamins and minerals) and ushering them out too.

Acetyl-L-Carnitine or L-Carnitine

Carnitine is essential for "carrying" free fatty acids into the mitochondrial energy production pipeline called *beta oxidation*; I have used this compound for years to treat both cognitive impairment and congestive heart failure patients. It is available in prescription form (as the drug Carnitor), but is also easily obtained as an over-the-counter supplement. I use acetyl-L-carnitine as part of my formula appropriately called Energy Renew for this ability. If pur-chasing, buy acetyl-L-carnitine 250 to 500 mg and take twice a day.

The Energy B Vitamins (Methyl B$_{12}$, Methyl Folate, and Vitamin B$_6$)

Since more than half the population carries one or more of the MTHFR mutations that prevent a complex action that otherwise makes several forms of vitamin B active in your body, I recom-mend supplementing daily with the active forms of B vitamins, methyl B$_{12}$ (1000 to 5000 mcg, under the tongue), methyl folate (1000 mcg), as well as vitamin B$_6$ in its active form, P-5-P (50 to 100 mg). Methyl B$_{12}$ is widely available—you can even find it at Costco. The complete range of the B vitamins are also contained in my powders, like Vital Reds, Primal Plants, and Power Blues.

Liver Protectors

A great number of my first-time patients suffer from fatty liver disease, or NASH or NAFLD, usually caused by a combination of mitochondrial overload, high fructose/sugar consumption, and leaky gut. If you have elevated liver enzymes, that is a sign that a literal war is being waged in your liver. I recommend the polyphe-nol milk thistle and a component of orange peel called d-limonene at a dose of about 1000 mg a day for both. They are remarkably ef-fective at reducing hepatic inflammation but are not an excuse for you to continue your previous eating behavior!

Berberine and Quercetin

Berberine, found in plants like bayberry and Oregon grape root (not to be confused with grape seed extract), and quercetin, found in foods such as onions, the pith of citrus fruits, and apples, are both compounds that have been shown to (among other things) activate a major driver of mitochondrial repair and mitogenesis called AMPK. The recommended dose of both is 500 mg twice a day. (By the way, for you allergy sufferers, quercetin is one of the best natural and non-sedating antihistamines available.)

Ketone Salts

Premade ketones are a great way to step up your game in ketone production. These can be swallowed in the form of salts or esters. To be quite frank, the esters taste pretty terrible, and I do not use or recommend them. On the other hand, ketone salts are readily available as powders or capsules and, early in the program, provide a usable boost in available ketones when you are not able to make them yourself because of elevated insulin levels. Consider a dose of about 10,000 mg mixed ketone salts (BHB) in the morning when starting the program. Think of it as a kick-start to having ketones circulating in your system until your body is able to produce your own.

The Energy Paradox G8

If you've read my previous books, you're already familiar with what I call the "G7s," which are the nutrients I strongly recommend incorporating into every diet—either through food or supplements—to support gut health, promote longevity, prevent disease, and enhance overall well-being. For the Energy Paradox Program, I've added one more essential nutrient to help boost overall energy production, so this list is now the "G8"! Without further ado, here are the eight supplements I want you to think about the next time you're filling your shopping cart at the grocery or health food store:

1. Vitamin D₃

Most patients who visit me are deficient in vitamin D, and all of my autoimmune, exhausted, and metabolically inflexible patients have low vitamin D levels. In fact, low vitamin D levels correlate strongly to metabolic syndrome as well as a susceptibility to COVID-19 and other viruses.[3] I recommend that everyone aim for a vitamin D level of 100–150 ng/ml (now considered "normal" by many labs including Quest and Cleveland HeartLab). While regular exposure to sunlight is one easy (and free) way to increase vitamin D production in the body, and foods such as mushrooms are abundant in this vitamin, both are insufficient to get you to the levels that are needed, in my opinion. When it comes to supplementation, I recommend a bare minimum of 5000 IUs (125 mcg) of vitamin D₃, but for my patients with leaky gut (and that's most of them), we start at 10,000 IUs (250 mcg).[4] I have yet to see vitamin D toxicity, even at levels of greater than 200 ng/ml, as confirmed by others as well.

2. Polyphenols

I'm constantly lecturing and publishing scientific papers about polyphenols—micronutrients found in certain plants—because they're incredible natural energy boosters and they provide so many other healing benefits. Polyphenols are great for heart health too: My own research has found that they improve blood vessel function and lower the markers for cardiovascular disease. They've also been shown to help balance healthy cholesterol levels. In addition, polyphenols feed the good bacteria in your gut, helping your body process more energy from food, and they enhance mitochondrial function by protecting against reactive oxygen species (ROS) generation during energy production.

Dark blue or purple fruits—like pomegranate, mulberries, Aronia berries, and dragon fruit—are very dense with polyphenols.

They're also found in many other food sources, including extra virgin olive oil, celery seed extract, turmeric, walnuts, capers, hazelnuts, coffee beans, ginger, tea, red wine, dark chocolate, endive, kale, and fennel seed.

3. Green Plant Phytochemicals

While your cravings for greens will increase exponentially on the Energy Paradox Program, I recommend taking phytochemicals in addition, as they tend to suppress your appetite for the unhealthy foods like simple sugars and fats.

There are many great blend powders on the market, but buyer beware: I have not been able to find a greens blend without wheat grass, barley grass, or oat grass as an ingredient (all gluten-containing lectins)—and the lectins in grains and grasses are the last things you need to swallow. I have my own green formula called Primal Plants that combines spinach extract with eleven other greens, particularly diindolylmethane (DIM), an immune-stimulating compound found in broccoli but in only small amounts, and modified citrus pectin and fructooligosaccharides (FOSs), the latter being an appetite suppressant and good for your gut buddies.

You could also take spinach extract, which is available in 500-mg capsules; I recommend you take two per day. DIM is available in capsule form; take 100 mg a day. I am also a big fan of modified citrus pectin, as it helps the body get rid of oxidative stress. It comes as a powder or in 600-mg capsules. Take two to three capsules or one scoop per day.

4. Prebiotics

You have read a lot about prebiotics in Part I, but it is worthwhile to give you specific recommendations if you want to ensure you are getting enough into your body. Inulin is readily available as a supplement or sweetener, while ground flaxseeds and/or psyllium powder are also easy to source. Start with a teaspoon a day and work up to about a tablespoon or more. I make my own PrebioThrive with multiple different prebiotic fibers—it is a convenient way to get several prebiotics at once.

5. Lectin Blockers

I admit, it's hard to stay away from lectins all the time. Luckily for you, a number of helpful compounds can help absorb them. Lectin Shield, one of my products, has nine proven ingredients to absorb or block them altogether from your gut wall. Before a lectin-containing meal, I suggest taking two capsules. You could also take glucosamine and methylsulfonylmethane (MSM) and/ or hyaluronic acid or a combo of all in tablet form. Products such as Osteo Bi-Flex and Move Free are available at Costco and other larger retailers.

6. Sugar Defenses

As you well know, sugar is everywhere, not only as table sugar, but also as high-fructose corn syrup and simple carbohydrates in your prepackaged foods and even in your favorite fruits. And this onslaught causes major issues for your energy-making mitochondria, who simply can't process all of that sugar at once. High sugar intake also interferes with insulin regulation, promoting insulin resistance and other metabolic problems, such as diabetes.

The most important thing you can do to protect yourself from sugar is to avoid eating it in the first place. But in addition to adjusting your diet, there are supplements that can help regulate your glucose, which will in turn lessen the traffic jam in your mitochondria. Look for a supplement that contains chromium, zinc, selenium, cinnamon bark extract, turmeric extract, berberine, and black pepper extract. (The latter enhances the absorbability of turmeric—anytime you consume turmeric, make sure you also consume black pepper!) Curcumin, the active ingredient in turmeric, is an antioxidant as well as an anti-inflammatory that also improves cognitive function. Costco sells a good chromium and cinnamon supplement called CinSulin. Take two capsules a day.

7. Long-Chain Omega-3s

Most people are profoundly deficient in the omega-3 fatty acids eicosapentaenoic acid (EPA) and, more important, docosahexaenoic acid (DHA) and docosapentaenoic acid (DPA). This is a problem because your brain is made up of approximately 60 percent fat, half of which is DHA. Studies show that people with the highest levels of omega-3 fats in their blood have a better memory and a bigger brain and better cognition than people with the lowest levels. You may also remember that fish oil helps repair your gut wall and keeps those nasty LPSs from leaking out into the rest of your body, where they generate energy-draining inflammation.

The only people in my practice who have sufficient levels of these brain-boosting fats without taking supplements are those who eat sardines or herring on a daily basis. Unless you're of Portuguese, Southern Italian, or Norwegian descent, you probably don't fit this profile, and you should supplement. I recommend choosing a fish oil that is molecularly distilled—there are several good national brands, like Nature's Bounty, OmegaVia, Carlson Elite Gems, or Carlson cod liver oil at a dose of a tablespoon a day. If you are vegan, select an algae-derived DHA, EPA, and DPA capsule like my Advanced Plant Omegas. Either way, aim to take 1000 mg of DHA per day, as it is the most important of the omega-3s, and, if you like, 1000 mg of EPA. At the time of this writing, there are reams of new research being published about the benefits of DPA, so stayed tuned for much more about this "forgotten" omega-3 fat.

8. Mitochondrial Boosters

Chrono consumption and exposure to red light are really the best ways to rev up your mitochondria, but for geeks like me, I also like to suggest a number of compounds to ensure you're doing the most you can for your ATP production. These include: N-acetyl L-cysteine (NAC), 500 mg; gynostemma extract, 450 mg; shilajit, 300 mg; reduced or L-glutathione, 150 mg; pau d'arco, 50 mg; and nicotinamide adenine dinucleotide, reduced (NADH), 10 mg.

When it comes to supplementing with NADH, there are several compounds available; one is nicotinamide riboside, patented and marketed as TRU Niagen. A recent human study suggested that a dose of 1000 mg a day raises the NAD+ level (an important precursor for ATP production in the mitochondria) in mononuclear cells. Not yet clinically available at a reasonable price (but certainly available) is nicotinamide mononucleotide at a similar dose, which my friend and fellow longevity researcher David Sinclair of Harvard Medical School and MIT has shown to be more efficacious than nicotinamide riboside in mouse trials. If cost is a concern, niacinamide, 500 to 1000 mg a day, is far more affordable and may, in fact, have the same effect.

AFTERWORD

When I began writing this book about the problem of persistent fatigue, we were living in a pre-pandemic world. A few months in, the COVID-19 virus emerged, began to rapidly spread around the globe, and our reality shifted dramatically. The challenges that resulted have been extraordinary in scope and scale and under the sustained conditions of stress and anxiety, energy levels have tipped further into the red. As I write these concluding words, we are still living with significant disruption to everyday life and uncertainty about the future—and, very sadly, many are grieving losses that nobody should have to face. Of loved ones, livelihoods, dreams, and ways of life. Perhaps even the loss of confidence in our ability to stay well.

Yet there are some things that I feel certain about: chief among them, your ability to boost your health by fortifying your gut, restoring conditions for a thriving microbiome, supplying your body with the nutrients that your immune system and your gut buddies require to do their jobs, and scheduling meals to ensure regular periods of cellular maintenance and repair. Over the long-term, taking these actions will help to build resilience against all kinds of unexpected invaders. Over the short-term, they will help you to restore your energy levels and feel like yourself again.

And guess what? That's exactly what you are doing by following the protocols in this book. Sure, you may have found aspects of the Energy Paradox Program a little challenging on first read. Perhaps the idea of changing your diet, your eating habits, or your habits of technology use, exercise, or sleep felt just a couple of degrees too extreme, especially now. But dear reader, at the risk of stating the obvious, these are extreme times. Though the exact mechanisms of how this virus (or the next one) operates are still coming into focus, this pandemic is showing us that the presumed benefits of our Western lifestyle have come with a terrible cost. Our immune systems are under assault, our protective microbiomes are decimated, and the pollution and chemicals we live with daily have made us uniquely vulnerable to a profound loss of energy, an epidemic of dementia and brain fog, chronic diseases like diabetes, and a seeming inability to defend against unwanted germs owing from these "preexisting conditions." The short takeaway: We have become sitting ducks, more vulnerable today than at any other time in recent history to pathogens like COVID-19.

But, through my years of practice, the wisdom that Hippocrates taught over 2,500 years ago—that all disease begins in the gut and that all creatures, including us, have an innate "green life force energy" or *veriditas*—has offered a different possibility. Through the guidance of my patients, I've learned that our bodies are well designed to not only keep us safe, but to thrive, if we give them (and our microbiome) what they need to achieve that goal. At the same time, we must remove the obstacles to it, including the disruptive conveniences that actually suppress veriditas. So, that starts with deciding right now to restore the conditions your veriditas requires, which will promote an optimally functioning immune system, which is funded by, you guessed it, plenty of energy.

The elders in our communities, including my recently departed parents, recall how their families rose to meet the extreme challenge of the Second World War by growing food at home—40 percent of our national food supply was grown in Victory gardens (while commodities like sugar and flour were rationed). This ensured food security and resiliency, but it also dramatically improved health markers as homegrown vegetables replaced insulin-spiking staples. Under today's unprecedented conditions of stay-at-home orders and restrictions, a similar movement is beginning to sprout as more of us regain connection to our food, whether by cooking it in our own kitchens, growing it ourselves, or sourcing it much closer to home. Paradoxical as it may seem, a new dawn *is* breaking out of this dark-seeming time, one in which we reclaim more agency over the very foundation of our health, starting with our food. By participating in the Paradox programs, by discovering new ways to feed yourself (and your gut buddies), you are part of this new beginning—regenerating our collective health from the ground up. My great hope is that this inspires you to walk with confidence, even while the terrain still feels uncertain.

ACKNOWLEDGMENTS

The Energy Paradox was written almost cover to cover during the COVID-19 pandemic, in starts and stops, during which I daily continued to see my full patient practice in person, both in Palm Springs and Santa Barbara, daily. And, as you can imagine, the writing process, even with collaboration from Amely Greeven and, late in the process, Kathy Huck, was laborious and halting, as concerns for family, staff, patients, safety precautions, and, well, lack of focus took its toll. But as I and others have said before, life doesn't happen to you, it happens *for* you. And in the case of *The Energy Paradox*, delays in actual time spent writing were gifts that allowed me to go down a few more rabbit holes to discover a few more gems that I hope amazed you as much as they fortified me, and strengthened this book. Thanks to both of you, Amely and Kathy!

The recipes were once again contributed by Kathryn "Kate" Holzhauer, my head chef at GundryMD, this time with some fun ways to get more gut-buddy-friendly foods into you, so they can make more postbiotics for your mitochondria. Delicious, Kate!

The team at HarperWave keeps going and going, but this time extreme thanks for the extra time you allowed to make this book one for the ages. I'm sure we will not forget what it took to bring this baby home. Of course, thanks to my publisher, Karen Rinaldi, VP of marketing Brian Perrin, publicity director Yelena Nesbit, art director Milan Bozic, who has designed all the Paradox covers, editorial assistant Emma Kupor, and, of course, vice president and editorial director Julie Will, who has been at the helm for all six of my bestsellers. It's a great team to have behind me and supporting me.

The team at the International Heart and Lung Institute and the Centers for Restorative Medicine in Palm Springs and Santa Barbara, California, stepped up to bat big-time with COVID-19 knocking on our doors. Led by my longtime executive assistant, Susan Lokken, and my now longtime colleague and physician's assistant, Mitsu Killion-Jacobo, our team of Adda Harris, Tanya Marta, Cindy Crosby, my daughter Melissa Perko, Yessenia Parra, and most-welcome newcomers, Nellie Melero and Erika Killion, all kept the doors open, safe, and welcoming all this time. Thank you again, from the bottom of my and, I'm sure, our patients' hearts. And the "blood suckers," Laurie Acuna, Lynn Visk, and Samantha Acuna, kept the blood tests flowing, despite risks.

Thanks also to my accountant Joe Tames and my attorney and friend Dave Baron, who keep the doors open.

All my work is guided by my longtime agent and early believer, Shannon Marven, president of Dupree Miller, who spent a lot of time on the phone begging for more time for me to get this book across the finish line during a pandemic. Thanks again, and can't wait for the "next one"!

Finally, I cannot express enough thanks to the six-hundred-plus people at GundryMD who have made me and GundryMD.com and *The Dr. Gundry Podcast* the trusted source for health and supplement advice for hundreds of millions of people daily. Despite the pandemic, a few of us arrive, screened and ready, every Friday at GundryMD, to bring you up-to-date information so vital to your health, especially now. And while I can't mention all of you here, thank you for continuing to service and support the millions of GundryMD family with our products and knowledge during this time. And again, a heartfelt thanks to my right-hand woman at GundryMD, Lanee Lee Neil, who protects and manages me, and, along with Kate mentioned above, my great team of writers, who keep the information flowing.

As I've said in all my Paradox books, nothing you read on any of these pages would be possible without my patients and my readers letting me learn from them over the last twenty years of practicing restorative medicine, which I continue to practice full-time six days a week (yes, even Saturday and Sunday). Thank you all again.

Finally, I wouldn't be able to do any of this without the love and support of my soul mate and wife, Penny. How she tolerates all this is astonishing! But, for those of you who asked about our destroyed house from the mudslides that I wrote about in *The Plant Paradox Family Cookbook*, life happens for you, not to you. We now have moved into a new house, which Penny, quite frankly, likes more than the destroyed one. Life, and energy, goes on!

APPENDIX:
LAB TESTS

When trying to assess your energy levels, the following are tests your health care provider can order. Your provider may be reluctant to order them because they simply don't know what they mean, but be persistent; they should know how important these are in measuring their patients' health. If your provider can't help or refuses to help, look for a restorative or functional medicine practitioner, many of whom can be found in your area by visiting www.ifm.org, the Institute for Functional Medicine.

I have not added values or markers to look for, because laboratories often use wildly different ranges and standards of test results.

Fasting Insulin and Insulin Resistance Score (sometimes called HOMA-IR)

Vitamin D level

Homocysteine

Fasting Glucose

HbA1C

Hs-CRP

Myeloperoxidase

TNF-alpha (if available)

Fibrinogen

Triglyceride/HDL ratio (HDL should be higher than triglycerides; if your triglycerides are above 80, you are overeating sugars and starches, including fruits)

Uric acid

Liver Function tests including GGT

Magnesium

Vitamin B_{12}

Serum folate

Calcium, serum

Zinc, serum

Selenium, serum

AM Cortisol

TSH (Thyroid-Stimulating Hormone)

Free T3

Free T4

Reverse T3

If taking thyroid hormones, order anti-TPO (Thyroperoxidase) and Antithyroglobulin levels as well, looking for markers of Hashimoto's autoimmune thyroiditis

Cystatin C (the "high-tech" way of measuring kidney function)

eGFR based on Cystatin C

NT-proBNP (a measurement of heart function)

NOTES

Chapter 1: How Did We Get Here?

1. Garton, Eric, "Employee Burnout Is a Problem with the Company, Not the Person," *Harvard Business Review*, July 20, 2017. https://hbr.org/2017/04/employee-burnout-is-a-problem-with-the-company-not-the-person.
2. Liu, Yun-Zi, Yun-Xia Wang, and Chun-Lei Jiang, "Inflammation: The Common Pathway of Stress-Related Diseases," *Frontiers*, June 1, 2017. https://www.frontiersin.org/articles/10.3389/fnhum.2017.00316/full.
3. "Stress Facts," Global Organization for Stress RSS. Accessed September 13, 2020. http://www.gostress.com/stress-facts/.
4. "45 Alarming Statistics on Americans' Caffeine Consumption," TheDiabetesCouncil.com. https://www.thediabetescouncil.com/45-alarming-statistics-on-americans-caffeine-consumption/.
5. Branum, Amy M., Lauren M. Rossen, and Kenneth C. Schoendorf, "Trends in Caffeine Intake Among US Children and Adolescents," *American Academy of Pediatrics*, March 1, 2014. https://pediatrics.aappublications.org/content/133/3/386.
6. Pontzer, Herman, et al., "Hunter-Gatherer Energetics and Human Obesity," *PLOS ONE*, July 25, 2012. https://journals.plos.org/plosone/article?id=10.1371%2Fjournal.pone.0040503.

Chapter 2: Body on Fire: How Inflammation Steals Your Energy

1. Wang, Hui, and Jianping Ye, "Regulation of Energy Balance by Inflammation: Common Theme in Physiology and Pathology," *Reviews in Endocrine & Metabolic Disorders* 16, no. 1 (2015): 47–54. doi:10.1007/s11154-014-9306-8.
2. Pontzer, Herman, et al., "Hunter-Gatherer Energetics and Human Obesity," *PLOS ONE*, July 25, 2012. https://www.ncbi.nlm.nih.gov/pmc/articles/PMC3405064/.
3. Amar, Jacques, et al., "Intestinal Mucosal Adherence and Translocation of Commensal Bacteria at the Early Onset of Type 2 Diabetes: Molecular Mechanisms and Probiotic Treatment," *EMBO Molecular Medicine*, John Wiley & Sons, Ltd, August 3, 2011. https://www.embopress.org/doi/abs/10.1002/emmm.201100159.
4. Gundry, Steven R., and Jean Epstein, "Abstract 137: Reversal of Endothelial Dysfunction Using Polyphenol Rich Foods and Supplements Coupled with Avoidance of Major Dietary Lectins," *Arteriosclerosis, Thrombosis, and Vascular Biology*, March 17, 2018. https://www.ahajournals.org/doi/abs/10.1161/atvb.33.suppl_1.a137.

Chapter 3: Damaged Roots, Degraded Soil, and the Postbiotic Conundrum

1. Verdam, Froukje J., et al., "Human Intestinal Microbiota Composition Is Associated with Local and Systemic Inflammation in Obesity," Wiley Online Library, John Wiley & Sons, Ltd, June 22, 2013. https://onlinelibrary.wiley.com/doi/pdf/10.1002/oby.20466.

2.   Fernández-Veledo, Sonia, and Joan Vendrell, "Gut Microbiota-Derived Succinate: Friend or Foe in Human Metabolic Diseases?" *Reviews in Endocrine and Metabolic Disorders*, Springer US, October 25, 2019. link.springer.com/article/10.1007/s11154-019-09513-z/figures/2.

3.   Smits, Samuel A., et al., "Seasonal Cycling in the Gut Microbiome of the Hadza Hunter-Gatherers of Tanzania," *Science*, American Association for the Advancement of Science, August 25, 2017. https://science.sciencemag.org/content/357/6353/802.full.

4.   Chiu, Karen, et al., "Impact of Environmental Chemicals on the Gut Microbiome," *OUP Academic*, Oxford University Press, May 11, 2020. https://academic.oup.com/toxsci/article/176/2/253/5835885.

5.   Patnode, Michael L., et al., "Interspecies Competition Impacts Targeted Manipulation of Human Gut Bacteria by Fiber-Derived Glycans," *Cell* 179, no. 1: 59–73.e13. doi: 10.1016/j.cell.2019.08.011.

6.   Nowak, Albina, MD, et. al., "Effect of Vitamin D_3 on Self-Perceived Fatigue," *Medicine* 95, no. 52 (December 2016): e5353. doi: 10.1097/MD.0000000000005353.

7.   Spiljar, Martina, Doron Merkler, and Mirko Trajkovski, "The Immune System Bridges the Gut Microbiota with Systemic Energy Homeostasis: Focus on TLRs, Mucosal Barrier, and SCFAs," *Frontiers*, October 3, 2017. https://www.frontiersin.org/articles/10.3389/fimmu.2017.01353/full.

8.   Rooks, Michelle G., and Wendy S. Garrett, "Gut Microbiota, Metabolites and Host Immunity," *Nature Reviews, Immunology*, U.S. National Library of Medicine, May 2016. https://pubmed.ncbi.nlm.nih.gov/27231050/.

9.   den Besten, Gijs, et al., "The Role of Short-Chain Fatty Acids in the Interplay between Diet, Gut Microbiota, and Host Energy Metabolism," *Journal of Lipid Research*, U.S. National Library of Medicine. Accessed September 13, 2020. https://pubmed.ncbi.nlm.nih.gov/23821742/.

10. den Besten, Gijs, et al., "Role of Short-Chain Fatty Acids."

11. Francis, C. Y., and P. J. Whorwell, "Bran and Irritable Bowel Syndrome: Time for Reappraisal," *Lancet* (London), U.S. National Library of Medicine, July 2, 1994. https://pubmed.ncbi.nlm.nih.gov/7912305/.

12. Leach, J. D., and K. D. Sobolik, "High Dietary Intake of Prebiotic Inulin-type Fructans in the Prehistoric Chihauhuan Desert," *British Journal of Nutrition*, 2010;103: 1158–61. https://pubmed.ncbi.nlm.nih.gov/20416127/, doi: 10.1017/S0007114510000966.

13. Barr, Sadie B., and Jonathan C. Wright, "Postprandial Energy Expenditure in Whole-Food and Processed-Food Meals: Implications for Daily Energy Expenditure," *Food & Nutrition Research*, U.S. National Library of Medicine, July 2, 2010. https://pubmed.ncbi.nlm.nih.gov/20613890/.

14. Zhang, C., "The Gut Flora-Centric Theory Based on the New Medical Hypothesis of 'Hunger Sensation Comes from Gut Flora': A New Model for Understanding the Etiology of Chronic Diseases in Human Beings," *Austin Internal Medicine* 3, no. 3 (2018). https://doi.org/10.26420/austin-intern-med.2018.1030.

15. Yan, Hui, and Kolapo M. Ajuwon, "Butyrate Modifies Intestinal Barrier Function in IPEC-J2 Cells through a Selective Upregulation of Tight Junction Proteins and Activation of the Akt Signaling Pathway," *PLOS ONE*, June 27, 2017. https://journals.plos.org/plosone/article?id=10.1371%2Fjournal.pone.0179586.

16. den Besten, Gijs, et al., "Role of Short-Chain Fatty Acids."

17. den Besten, Gijs, et al., "Gut-Derived Short-Chain Fatty Acids Are Vividly Assimilated into Host Carbohydrates and Lipids." *The American Journal of Physiology-Gastrointestinal and Liver Physiology* 305, no. 12. U.S. National Library of Medicine. December 2013. https://pubmed.ncbi.nlm.nih.gov/24136789/.

18. Chang, Pamela V., et al., "The Microbial Metabolite Butyrate Regulates Intestinal Macrophage Function via Histone Deacetylase Inhibition," *PNAS*, National Academy of Sciences, February 11, 2014. https://www.pnas.org/content/111/6/2247.

19. Hylemon, Phillip B., Spencer C. Harris, and Jason M. Ridlon, "Metabolism of Hydrogen Gases and Bile Acids in the Gut Microbiome," *FEBS Press*, John Wiley & Sons, Ltd, May 7, 2018. https://febs.onlinelibrary.wiley.com/doi/full/10.1002/1873-3468.13064.

20. McNabney, Sean M., and Tara Henagan, "Short Chain Fatty Acids in the Colon and Peripheral Tissues: A Focus on Butyrate, Colon Cancer, Obesity and Insulin Resistance," *Nutrients* 9, no. 12 (2017): 1348. https://doi.org/10.3390/nu9121348.

21. Barrea, Luigi, et al., "From Gut Microbiota Dysfunction to Obesity: Could Short-Chain Fatty Acids Stop This Dangerous Course?" *Hormones* (Athens, Greece), U.S. National Library of Medicine, March 6, 2019. https://pubmed.ncbi.nlm.nih.gov/30840230.

22. Goh, Charlene E., et al., "Association Between Nitrate-Reducing Oral Bacteria and Cardiometabolic Outcomes: Results From ORIGINS," *Journal of the American Heart Association*, November 26, 2019. https://www.ahajournals.org/doi/10.1161/JAHA.119.013324.

23. Nicholls, Mark, "Nitric Oxide Discovery Nobel Prize Winners: Robert F. Furchgott, Louis J. Ignarro, and Ferid Murad Shared the Noble Prize in 1998 for Their Discoveries Concerning Nitric Oxide as a Signalling Molecule in the Cardiovascular System," *OUP Academic*, Oxford University Press, June 7, 2019. https://academic.oup.com/eurheartj/article/40/22/1747/5512074.

24. Case Western Reserve University, "New 'Interspecies Communication' Strategy between Gut Bacteria and Mammalian Hosts Uncovered," Phys.org, February 21, 2019. https://phys.org/news/2019-02-interspecies-strategy-gut-bacteria-mammalian.html.

25. Mészáros, András Tamás, et al., "Mitochondria as Sources and Targets of Methane," *Frontiers*, October 25, 2017. https://www.frontiersin.org/articles/10.3389/fmed.2017.00195/full.

26. Altaany, Zaid, et al., "Evaluation of Antioxidant Status and Oxidative Stress Markers in Thermal Sulfurous Springs Residents," *Heliyon*, Elsevier, November 29, 2019. https://www.sciencedirect.com/science/article/pii/S2405844019365442.

27. Ostojic, Sergej M., "Inadequate Production of H_2 by Gut Microbiota and Parkinson Disease," *Trends in Endocrinology and Metabolism*, U.S. National Library of Medicine, May 2018. https://pubmed.ncbi.nlm.nih.gov/29478695/.

28. Scheperjans, Filip, et al., "Gut Microbiota Are Related to Parkinson's Disease and Clinical Phenotype," *Movement Disorders: Official Journal of the Movement Disorder Society*, U.S. National Library of Medicine, March 2015. https://pubmed.ncbi.nlm.nih.gov/25476529/.

29. Niu, Yinghao, et al., "Hydrogen Attenuates Allergic Inflammation by Reversing Energy Metabolic Pathway Switch," *Nature News*, Nature Publishing Group, February 6, 2020. https://www.nature.com/articles/s41598-020-58999-0.

30. Han, Yuyi, et al., "Hydrogen Sulfide: A Gaseous Signaling Molecule Modulates Tissue Homeostasis: Implications in Ophthalmic Diseases," *Cell Death & Disease*, Nature Publishing Group, March 29, 2019. https://www.nature.com/articles/s41419-019-1525-1.

31. Shefa, Ulfuara, et al., "Roles of Gasotransmitters in Synaptic Plasticity and Neuropsychiatric Conditions," *Neural Plasticity*, Hindawi, May 6, 2018. https://www.hindawi.com/journals/np/2018/1824713/.

32. Lu, Ming, et al., "Hydrogen Sulfide Inhibits Plasma Renin Activity," *Journal of the American Society of Nephrology*, June 21, 2010. https://www.ncbi.nlm.nih.gov/pmc/articles/PMC2900962/.

33. Peh, Meng Teng, et al., "Effect of Feeding a High-Fat Diet on Hydrogen Sulfide (H_2S)

Metabolism in the Mouse," *Nitric Oxide*, Academic Press, March 14, 2014. https://www
.sciencedirect.com/science/article/pii/S1089860314000226.

34. Peh, Meng Teng, et al., "Effect of Feeding a High-Fat Diet."

35. Xie, Zhi-Zhong, Yang Liu, and Jin-Song Bian, "Hydrogen Sulfide and Cellular Redox
Homeostasis," *Oxidative Medicine and Cellular Longevity*, Hindawi, January 5, 2016.
https://www.hindawi.com/journals/omcl/2016/6043038/.

36. Szabo, Csaba, et al., "Regulation of Mitochondrial Bioenergetic Function by Hydrogen
Sulfide. Part I. Biochemical and Physiological Mechanisms," *British Journal of Pharmacology* 171, no. 8 (2014): 2099–122. https://doi.org/10.1111/bph.12369.

37. Fu, Ming, et al., "Hydrogen Sulfide (H_2S) Metabolism in Mitochondria and Its Regulatory Role in Energy Production," *Proceedings of the National Academy of Sciences*,
National Academy of Sciences, February 21, 2012. https://www.ncbi.nlm.nih.gov/pmc
/articles/PMC3287003.

38. Guo, Wei, et al., "Hydrogen Sulfide as an Endogenous Modulator in Mitochondria and
Mitochondria Dysfunction," *Oxidative Medicine and Cellular Longevity* 2012 (December 5, 2012): 1–9. https://doi.org/10.1155/2012/878052.

39. Sonnenburg, Justin L., and Fredrik Bäckhed, "Diet-Microbiota Interactions as Mod-
erators of Human Metabolism," *Nature News*, Nature Publishing Group, July 6, 2016.
https://www.nature.com/articles/nature18846.

40. Cohen, S., et al., "Chronic Stress, Glucocorticoid Receptor Resistance, Inflammation,
and Disease Risk," *Proceedings of the National Academy of Sciences* 109, no. 16 (2012):
5995–99. https://doi.org/10.1073/pnas.1118355109.

Chapter 4: Your Mighty Mitochondria Are All Mixed Up

1. "Mitochondrial Dysfunction Is the Root Cause of Many Diseases," *ScienceDaily*, January 26, 2017. https://www.sciencedaily.com/releases/2017/01/170126093255.htm.

2. Rich, Peter, "Chemiosmotic Coupling: The Cost of Living," *Nature News*, Nature Publishing Group. Accessed September 11, 2020. https://www.nature.com/articles/421583a.

3. Degli Esposti, Mauro, "Bioenergetic Evolution in Proteobacteria and Mitochondria,"
Genome Biology and Evolution, Oxford University Press, November 27, 2014. https://
www.ncbi.nlm.nih.gov/pmc/articles/PMC4986455/.

4. Guo, Chunyan, et al., "Oxidative Stress, Mitochondrial Damage and Neurodegenerative Diseases," *Neural Regeneration Research*, Medknow Publications & Media Pvt Ltd,
July 25, 2013. https://www.ncbi.nlm.nih.gov/pmc/articles/PMC4145906/.

5. Kundu, P., et al., "Neurogenesis and Prolongevity Signaling in Young Germ-Free Mice
Transplanted with the Gut Microbiota of Old Mice," *Science Translational Medicine*, U.S.
National Library of Medicine, pubmed.ncbi.nlm.nih.gov/31723038/.

6. Muoio, Deborah M., "Metabolic Inflexibility: When Mitochondrial Indecision Leads
to Metabolic Gridlock," *Cell* 159, no. 6 (2014): 1253–62. https://doi.org/10.1016/j.cell
.2014.11.034.

7. Sommer, Andrei P., Mike Kh. Haddad, and Hans-Jörg Fecht, "Light Effect on Water
Viscosity: Implication for ATP Biosynthesis," *Scientific Reports*, Nature Publishing
Group, July 8, 2015. https://www.ncbi.nlm.nih.gov/pmc/articles/PMC4495567/.

8. Pannala, Venkat R., Amadou K. Camara, and Ranjan K. Dash, "Modeling the Detailed
Kinetics of Mitochondrial Cytochrome c Oxidase: Catalytic Mechanism and Nitric
Oxide Inhibition," *Journal of Applied Physiology* (Bethesda, MD: 1985), U.S. National
Library of Medicine. https://pubmed.ncbi.nlm.nih.gov/27633738/.

9. Herrera, Arturo Solis, "Melanin, Energy and the Cell," *Diabetes & Obesity International
Journal* 2, no. S1 (2017). https://doi.org/10.23880/doij-16000s1-004.

10. Ball, Writoban Basu, John K. Neff, and Vishal M. Gohil, "The Role of Nonbilayer Phospholipids in Mitochondrial Structure and Function," *FEBS Press*, John Wiley & Sons,

Ltd, November 9, 2017. https://febs.onlinelibrary.wiley.com/doi/full/10.1002/1873
-3468.12887.

11.   Sullivan, E. Madison, et al., "Mechanisms by Which Dietary Fatty Acids Regulate
      Mitochondrial Structure-Function in Health and Disease," *Advances in Nutrition*
      (Bethesda, MD), U.S. National Library of Medicine, May 1, 2018. https://pubmed.ncbi
      .nlm.nih.gov/29767698.

12.   Høy, C.-E., et al., "Incorporation of Cis- and Trans-Octadecenoic Acids into the Mem-
      branes of Rat Liver Mitochondria," *Lipids*, Springer-Verlag, January 1, 1969. https://
      link.springer.com/article/10.1007/BF02533898.

13.   "Melatonin Protects the Powerhouses of Cells, the Mitochondria," *Atlas of Science*.
      Accessed September 11, 2020. https://atlasofscience.org/melatonin-protects-the
      -powerhouses-of-cells-the-mitochondria/.

14.   Zimmerman, Scott, and Russel J. Reiter, "Melatonin and the Optics of the Human
      Body," *Melatonin Research*, 2019. https://www.researchgate.net/publication/331410779
      _Melatonin_and_the_Optics_of_the_Human_Body.

15.   Contrepois, Kévin, et al., "Molecular Choreography of Acute Exercise," *Cell Press*,
      May 28, 2020. https://doi.org/10.1016/j.cell.2020.04.043.

16.   Chaurasia, Bhagirath, and Scott A. Summers, "Ceramides—Lipotoxic Inducers of
      Metabolic Disorders," *Trends in Endocrinology & Metabolism* 26, no. 10 (2015): 538–50.
      https://doi.org/10.1016/j.tem.2015.07.006.

17.   Peterson, Linda R., et al., "Ceramide Remodeling and Risk of Cardiovascular Events
      and Mortality," *Journal of the American Heart Association* 7, no. 10 (2018). doi:10.1161
      /jaha.117.007931.

18.   Butler, T. J., et al., "Western Diet Increases Cardiac Ceramide Content in Healthy and
      Hypertrophied Hearts," *Nutrition, Metabolism and Cardiovascular Diseases* 27, no. 11
      (2017): 991–98. doi:10.1016/j.numecd.2017.08.007.

19.   Tharyan, Rebecca George, et al., "NFYB-1 Regulates Mitochondrial Function and
      Longevity via Lysosomal Prosaposin," *Nature Metabolism* 2, no. 5 (2020): 387–96.
      https://doi.org/10.1038/s42255-020-0200-2.

20.   Law, Brittany A., et al., "Lipotoxic Very-Long-Chain Ceramides Cause Mitochondrial
      Dysfunction, Oxidative Stress, and Cell Death in Cardiomyocytes," *FASEB Journal* 32,
      no. 3 (2018): 1403–16. https://doi.org/10.1096/fj.201700300r.

21.   Sokolowska, Emilia, and Agnieszka Blachnio-Zabielska, "The Role of Ceramides in
      Insulin Resistance," *Frontiers*, August 7, 2019. https://www.frontiersin.org/articles
      /10.3389/fendo.2019.00577/full.

22.   Pinel, Alexandre, et al., "N - 3PUFA Differentially Modulate Palmitate-Induced Li-
      potoxicity through Alterations of Its Metabolism in C2C12 Muscle Cells," *Biochimica
      et Biophysica Acta (BBA)—Molecular and Cell Biology of Lipids*, Elsevier, October 22, 2015.
      https://www.sciencedirect.com/science/article/abs/pii/S1388198115001912.

23.   Parker, Brian A., et al., "β-Hydroxybutyrate Elicits Favorable Mitochondrial Changes
      in Skeletal Muscle," *International Journal of Molecular Sciences*, MDPI, August 1, 2018.
      https://www.ncbi.nlm.nih.gov/pmc/articles/PMC6121962.

24.   Chinopoulos, Christos, and Vera Adam-Vizi, "Mitochondria as ATP Consumers in
      Cellular Pathology," *Biochimica et Biophysica Acta*, U.S. National Library of Medicine,
      January 2010. https://pubmed.ncbi.nlm.nih.gov/19715757.

Chapter 5: Inflamed and Energy Starved: The Tired Modern Brain

1.   Thompson, Robert S., et al., "Dietary Prebiotics Alter Novel Microbial Dependent Fe-
      cal Metabolites That Improve Sleep," *Nature News*, Nature Publishing Group, March 2,
      2020. https://www.nature.com/articles/s41598-020-60679-y.

2.   Zhu, Xiao-Hong, et al., "Quantitative Imaging of Energy Expenditure in Human

Brain," *NeuroImage* 60, no. 4 (2012): 2107–17. https://doi.org/10.1016/j.neuroimage .2012.02.013.

3. Yarandi, Shadi S., et al., "Modulatory Effects of Gut Microbiota on the Central Nervous System: How Gut Could Play a Role in Neuropsychiatric Health and Diseases," *Journal of Neurogastroenterology and Motility* 22, no. 2 (2016): 201–12. https://doi.org/10.5056 /jnm15146.

4. Mayer, Emeran A., David Padua, and Kirsten Tillisch, "Altered Brain-Gut Axis in Autism: Comorbidity or Causative Mechanisms?" *BioEssays: News and Reviews in Molecular, Cellular and Developmental Biology*, U.S. National Library of Medicine, August 22, 2014. https://pubmed.ncbi.nlm.nih.gov/25145752/.

5. de Theije, Caroline G. M., et al., "Altered Gut Microbiota and Activity in a Murine Model of Autism Spectrum Disorders," *Brain, Behavior, and Immunity* 37 (2014): 197–206. https://doi.org/10.1016/j.bbi.2013.12.005.

6. Severance, Emily G., et al., "Discordant Patterns of Bacterial Translocation Markers and Implications for Innate Immune Imbalances in Schizophrenia," *Schizophrenia Research*, U.S. National Library of Medicine, June 6, 2013. https://pubmed.ncbi.nlm.nih .gov/23746484/.

7. Steenbergen, Laura, et al., "A Randomized Controlled Trial to Test the Effect of Multi-species Probiotics on Cognitive Reactivity to Sad Mood," *Brain, Behavior, and Immunity* 48 (2015): 258–64. https://doi.org/10.1016/j.bbi.2015.04.003.

8. Valles-Colomer, Mireia, et al., "The Neuroactive Potential of the Human Gut Microbiota in Quality of Life and Depression," *Nature Microbiology* 4, no. 4 (2019): 623–32. https://doi.org/10.1038/s41564-018-0337-x.

9. Sun, Yayi, et al., "Intra-Gastrointestinal Amyloid-β1–42 Oligomers Perturb Enteric Function and Induce Alzheimer's Disease Pathology," *Journal of Physiology*, July 2, 2020. https://doi.org/10.1113/jp279919.

10. Noonan, Sanjay, et al., "Food & Mood: A Review of Supplementary Prebiotic and Probiotic Interventions in the Treatment of Anxiety and Depression in Adults," *BMJ Nutrition, Prevention & Health*, 2020. https://doi.org/10.1136/bmjnph-2019-000053.

11. Noble, Emily E., Ted M. Hsu, and Scott E. Kanoski, "Gut to Brain Dysbiosis: Mechanisms Linking Western Diet Consumption, the Microbiome, and Cognitive Impairment," *Frontiers in Behavioral Neuroscience* 11 (2017). https://doi.org/10.3389/fnbeh .2017.00009.

12. Bonaz, Bruno, Thomas Bazin, and Sonia Pellissier, "The Vagus Nerve at the Interface of the Microbiota-Gut-Brain Axis," *Frontiers in Neuroscience* 12 (2018). https://doi .org/10.3389/fnins.2018.00049.

13. Obrenovich, Mark E. M., "Leaky Gut, Leaky Brain?" *MDPI*, Multidisciplinary Digital Publishing Institute, October 18, 2018. https://www.mdpi.com/2076-2607/6/4/107.

14. Noble, Emily E., et al., "Gut to Brain Dysbiosis."

15. Martinez, Adriana, and Abraham J. Al-Ahmad, "Effects of Glyphosate and Amino-methylphosphonic Acid on an Isogeneic Model of the Human Blood-Brain Barrier." *Comparative Study Toxicol Lett*, April 2019. https://www.ncbi.nlm.nih.gov/pubmed/30605748.

16. Morley, Wendy A., and Stephanie Seneff, "Diminished Brain Resilience Syndrome: A Modern Day Neurological Pathology of Increased Susceptibility to Mild Brain Trauma, Concussion, and Downstream Neurodegeneration," *Surgical Neurology International* 5, no. 1 (2014): 97. https://doi.org/10.4103/2152-7806.134731.

17. Schinkel, Alfred H., "P-Glycoprotein, a Gatekeeper in the Blood-Brain Barrier," *Advanced Drug Delivery Reviews* 36 (1999): 179–94.

18. Wadhwa, Meetu, et al., "Inhibiting the Microglia Activation Improves the Spatial Memory and Adult Neurogenesis in Rat Hippocampus during 48 h of Sleep Depriva-

tion," *Journal of Neuroinflammation*, BioMed Central, January 1, 1970. https://jneuro inflammation.biomedcentral.com/articles/10.1186/s12974-017-0998-z.

19. Liu, Yun-Zi, Yun-Xia Wang, and Chun-Lei Jiang, "Inflammation: The Common Pathway of Stress-Related Diseases," *Frontiers in Human Neuroscience* 11 (2017). https://doi .org/10.3389/fnhum.2017.00316.

20. van Kessel, Sebastiaan, and Sahar El Aidy, "Bacterial Metabolites Mirror Altered Gut Microbiota Composition in Patients with Parkinson's Disease," *Journal of Parkinson's Disease* 9, no. s2 (2019). https://doi.org/10.3233/jpd-191780.

21. Wu, Xinwei, et al., "Hydrogen Exerts Neuroprotective Effects on OGD/R Damaged Neurons in Rat Hippocampal by Protecting Mitochondrial Function via Regulating Mitophagy Mediated by PINK1/Parkin Signaling Pathway," *Brain Research* 1698 (2018): 89–98. https://doi.org/10.1016/j.brainres.2018.06.028.

22. Bourassa, Megan W., et al., "Butyrate, Neuroepigenetics and the Gut Microbiome: Can a High Fiber Diet Improve Brain Health?" *Neuroscience Letters* 625 (2016): 56–63. https://doi.org/10.1016/j.neulet.2016.02.009.

23. Kundu, Parag, et al., "Neurogenesis and Prolongevity Signaling in Young Germ-Free Mice Transplanted with the Gut Microbiota of Old Mice," *Science Translational Medicine* 11, no. 518 (2019). https://doi.org/10.1126/scitranslmed.aau4760.

24. Erny, Daniel, et al., "Host Microbiota Constantly Control Maturation and Function of Microglia in the CNS," *Nature Neuroscience* 18, no. 7 (2015): 965–77. https://doi.org /10.1038/nn.4030.

25. Khan, Naiman A., et al., "Dietary Fiber Is Positively Associated with Cognitive Control among Prepubertal Children," *The Journal of Nutrition* 145, no. 1 (2014): 143–49. https://doi.org/10.3945/jn.114.198457.

26. Wu, Xinwei, et al., "Hydrogen Exerts Neuroprotective Effects."

27. Dalile, Boushra, et al., "The Role of Short-Chain Fatty Acids in Microbiota-Gut-Brain Communication," *Nature Reviews Gastroenterology & Hepatology*, 16(8): 461–78, U.S. National Library of Medicine, August 2019. https://pubmed.ncbi.nlm.nih.gov /31123355.

28. Klinedinst, Brandon S., et al., "Aging-Related Changes in Fluid Intelligence, Muscle and Adipose Mass, and Sex-Specific Immunologic Mediation: A Longitudinal UK Biobank Study," *Brain, Behavior, and Immunity* 82 (2019): 396–405. https://doi.org /10.1016/j.bbi.2019.09.008.

29. Mielke, M. M., et al., "Serum Ceramides Increase the Risk of Alzheimer Disease: The Women's Health and Aging Study II," *Neurology* 79, no. 7 (2012): 633–41. https://doi .org/10.1212/wnl.0b013e318264e380.

30. Liu, Yun-Zi, Yun-Xia Wang, and Chun-Lei Jiang, "Inflammation: The Common Pathway of Stress-Related Diseases."

31. Galland, Leo, "The Gut Microbiome and the Brain," *Journal of Medicinal Food* 17, no. 12 (2014): 1261–72. https://doi.org/10.1089/jmf.2014.7000.

32. Guenther, G. G., et al., "Ceramide Starves Cells to Death by Downregulating Nutrient Transporter Proteins," *Proceedings of the National Academy of Sciences* 105, no. 45 (2008): 17402–7. https://doi.org/10.1073/pnas.0802781105.

33. Carr, Sheryl Teresa, "Insulin and Ketones: Their Roles in Brain Mitochondrial Function," BYU Scholars Archive, Brigham Young University, 2017. https://scholarsarchive .byu.edu/etd/6810.

34. Xu, Youhua, Hua Zhou, and Quan Zhu, "The Impact of Microbiota-Gut-Brain Axis on Diabetic Cognition Impairment," *Frontiers in Aging Neuroscience* 9 (2017). https://doi .org/10.3389/fnagi.2017.00106.

35. Martínez-Lapiscina, Elena H., et al., "Mediterranean Diet Improves Cognition: the

PREDIMED-NAVARRA Randomised Trial," *Journal of Neurology, Neurosurgery & Psychiatry* 84, no. 12 (2013): 1318–25. https://doi.org/10.1136/jnnp-2012-304792.

36. Noble, Emily E., et al., "Gut to Brain Dysbiosis."

Chapter 6: It's All about Timing (and Good Choices)

1. de Cabo, Rafael, and Mark P. Mattson, "Effects of Intermittent Fasting on Health, Aging, and Disease," *New England Journal of Medicine* 381, no. 26 (2019): 2541–51. https://doi.org/10.1056/nejmra1905136.

2. Cignarella, Francesca, et al., "Intermittent Fasting Confers Protection in CNS Autoimmunity by Altering the Gut Microbiota," *Cell Metabolism* 27, no. 6 (2018). https://doi.org/10.1016/j.cmet.2018.05.006.

3. Zarrinpar, Amir, et al., "Diet and Feeding Pattern Affect the Diurnal Dynamics of the Gut Microbiome," *Cell Metabolism* 20, no. 6 (2014): 1006–17. https://doi.org/10.1016/j.cmet.2014.11.008.

4. Chaix, Amandine, et al., "Time-Restricted Eating to Prevent and Manage Chronic Metabolic Diseases," *Annual Review of Nutrition* 39, no. 1 (2019): 291–315. https://doi.org/10.1146/annurev-nutr-082018-124320.

5. Stekovic, Slaven, et al., "Alternate Day Fasting Improves Physiological and Molecular Markers of Aging in Healthy, Non-Obese Humans," *Cell Metabolism* 30, no. 3 (2019). https://doi.org/10.1016/j.cmet.2019.07.016.

6. Mitchell, Sarah J., et al., "Daily Fasting Improves Health and Survival in Male Mice Independent of Diet Composition and Calories," *Cell Metabolism* 29, no. 1 (2019). https://doi.org/10.1016/j.cmet.2018.08.011.

7. Moro, Tatiana, et al., "Effects of Eight Weeks of Time-Restricted Feeding (16/8) on Basal Metabolism, Maximal Strength, Body Composition, Inflammation, and Cardiovascular Risk Factors in Resistance-Trained Males," *Journal of Translational Medicine* 14, no. 1 (2016). https://doi.org/10.1186/s12967-016-1044-0.

8. Chaix, Amandine, et al., "Time-Restricted Feeding Is a Preventative and Therapeutic Intervention against Diverse Nutritional Challenges," *Cell Metabolism* 20, no. 6 (2014): 991–1005. doi: 10.1016/j.cmet.2014.11.001.

9. Monique Tello, "Intermittent Fasting: Surprising Update," *Harvard Health* blog, February 10, 2020. https://www.health.harvard.edu/blog/intermittent-fasting-surprising-update-2018062914156.

10. Brown, Andrew W., Michelle M. Bohan Brown, and David B. Allison, "Belief beyond the Evidence: Using the Proposed Effect of Breakfast on Obesity to Show 2 Practices That Distort Scientific Evidence," *American Journal of Clinical Nutrition* 98, no. 5 (2013): 1298–1308. https://doi.org/10.3945/ajcn.113.064410.

11. Matheson, Paul J., Mark A. Wilson, and R. Neal Garrison, "Regulation of Intestinal Blood Flow," *Journal of Surgical Research* 93, no. 1 (2000): 182–96. https://doi.org/10.1006/jsre.2000.5862.

12. Wallis, Gareth A., and Javier T. Gonzalez, "Is Exercise Best Served on an Empty Stomach?" *Proceedings of the Nutrition Society*, U.S. National Library of Medicine, October 18, 2018. https://pubmed.ncbi.nlm.nih.gov/30334499/.

13. Chavan, Rohit, et al., "Liver-Derived Ketone Bodies Are Necessary for Food Anticipation," *Nature Communications* 7, no. 1 (2016). https://doi.org/10.1038/ncomms10580.

14. Chavan, Rohit, et al. "Liver-Derived Ketone Bodies Are Necessary for Food Anticipation." *Nature Communications*, Nature Publishing Group. February 3, 2016. www.ncbi.nlm.nih.gov/pmc/articles/PMC4742855/.

15. Longo, Valter D., and Satchidananda Panda, "Fasting, Circadian Rhythms, and Time-Restricted Feeding in Healthy Lifespan," *Cell Metabolism* 23, no. 6 (2016): 1048–59. https://doi.org/10.1016/j.cmet.2016.06.001.

16. Mindikoglu, Ayse L., et al., "Intermittent Fasting from Dawn to Sunset for 30 Consecutive Days Is Associated with Anticancer Proteomic Signature and Upregulates Key Regulatory Proteins of Glucose and Lipid Metabolism, Circadian Clock, DNA Repair, Cytoskeleton Remodeling, Immune System and Cognitive Function in Healthy Subjects," *Journal of Proteomics* 217 (2020): 103645. https://doi.org/10.1016/j.jprot.2020.103645.

17. Rahbar, Alir, et al., "Effects of Intermittent Fasting during Ramadan on Insulin-like Growth Factor-1, Interleukin 2, and Lipid Profile in Healthy Muslims," *International Journal of Preventive Medicine* 10, no. 1 (2019): 7. https://doi.org/10.4103/ijpvm.ijpvm_252_17.

18. Gill, Shubhroz, and Satchidananda Panda, "A Smartphone App Reveals Erratic Diurnal Eating Patterns in Humans That Can Be Modulated for Health Benefits," *Cell Metabolism* 22, no. 5 (2015): 789–98. https://doi.org/10.1016/j.cmet.2015.09.005.

19. Wahl, Devin, et al., "Cognitive and Behavioral Evaluation of Nutritional Interventions in Rodent Models of Brain Aging and Dementia," *Clinical Interventions in Aging* 12 (2017): 1419–28. https://doi.org/10.2147/cia.S145247.

20. Schmitt, Karen, et al., "Circadian Control of DRP1 Activity Regulates Mitochondrial Dynamics and Bioenergetics," *Cell Metabolism* 27, no. 3 (2018). https://doi.org/10.1016/j.cmet.2018.01.011.

21. Newman, John C., and Eric Verdin, "Ketone Bodies as Signaling Metabolites," *Trends in Endocrinology & Metabolism* 25, no. 1 (2014): 42–52. https://doi.org/10.1016/j.tem.2013.09.002.

22. de Cabo, Rafael, and Mark P. Mattson, "Effects of Intermittent Fasting on Health, Aging, and Disease."

23. Luna-Sánchez, Marta, et al., "CoQ Deficiency Causes Disruption of Mitochondrial Sulfide Oxidation, a New Pathomechanism Associated with this Syndrome," *EMBO Molecular Medicine* 9, no. 1 (2016): 78–95. https://doi.org/10.15252/emmm.201606345.

24. Hine, Christopher, and James R. Mitchell, "Calorie Restriction and Methionine Restriction in Control of Endogenous Hydrogen Sulfide Production by the Transsulfuration Pathway," *Experimental Gerontology* 68 (2015): 26–32. https://doi.org/10.1016/j.exger.2014.12.010.

25. Perridon, Bernard W., et al., "The Role of Hydrogen Sulfide in Aging and Age-Related Pathologies," *Aging*, Impact Journals LLC, September 27, 2016. https://www.ncbi.nlm.nih.gov/pmc/articles/PMC5115888.

26. Li, Shuanshuang, and Guandong Yang, "Hydrogen Sulfide Maintains Mitochondrial DNA Replication via Demethylation of TFAM," *Antioxidants & Redox Signaling*, U.S. National Library of Medicine, May 14, 2015. https://pubmed.ncbi.nlm.nih.gov/25758951.

27. Zhang, Hongbo, Keir J. Menzies, and Johan Auwerx, "The Role of Mitochondria in Stem Cell Fate and Aging," *Development* 145, no. 8 (2018). https://doi.org/10.1242/dev.143420.

28. Ruiz, Atenodoro R., "Carbohydrate Intolerance—Gastrointestinal Disorders," Merck Manuals Professional Edition, Merck Manuals. Content last modified October 2019. Accessed September 13, 2020. https://www.merckmanuals.com/professional/gastrointestinal-disorders/malabsorption-syndromes/carbohydrate-intolerance.

29. Greenhill, Claire, "Ketogenic Diet Affects Immune Cells in Mice," *Nature Reviews Endocrinology* 16, no. 4 (2020): 196–97. https://doi.org/10.1038/s41574-020-0328-x.

30. Goldberg, Emily L., et al., "Ketogenesis Activates Metabolically Protective γδT Cells in Visceral Adipose Tissue," *Nature Metabolism* 2, no. 1 (2020): 50–61. https://www.nature.com/articles/s42255-019-0160-6.

31. Edwards, Lindsay M., et al., "Short-Term Consumption of a High-Fat Diet Impairs Whole-Body Efficiency and Cognitive Function in Sedentary Men," *FASEB Journal* 25, no. 3 (2010): 1088–96. https://doi.org/10.1096/fj.10-171983.

32. Miller, Vincent J., Frederick A. Villamena, and Jeff S. Volek, "Nutritional Ketosis and Mitohormesis: Potential Implications for Mitochondrial Function and Human Health," *Journal of Nutrition and Metabolism* 2018: 1–27. https://doi.org/10.1155/2018/5157645.

33. Bak, Ann Mosegaard, et al., "Prolonged Fasting-Induced Metabolic Signatures in Human Skeletal Muscle of Lean and Obese Men," *PLOS ONE* 13, no. 9 (2018). https://doi.org/10.1371/journal.pone.0200817.

34. Groennebaek, Thomas, and Kristian Vissing, "Impact of Resistance Training on Skeletal Muscle Mitochondrial Biogenesis, Content, and Function," *Frontiers in Physiology* 8 (2017). https://doi.org/10.3389/fphys.2017.00713.

35. Van Proeyen, Karen, et al., "Training in the Fasted State Improves Glucose Tolerance during Fat-Rich Diet," *Journal of Physiology*, U.S. National Library of Medicine, November 2010. https://pubmed.ncbi.nlm.nih.gov/20837645/.

36. Contrepois, Kévin, et al., "Molecular Choreography of Acute Exercise," *Cell* 181, no. 5 (2020). https://doi.org/10.1016/j.cell.2020.04.043.

37. Liu, Yan, et al., "Gut Microbiome Fermentation Determines the Efficacy of Exercise for Diabetes Prevention," *Cell Metabolism* 31, no. 1 (2020). https://doi.org/10.1016/j.cmet.2019.11.001.

38. Glynn, Erin L., et al., "Impact of Combined Resistance and Aerobic Exercise Training on Branched-Chain Amino Acid Turnover, Glycine Metabolism and Insulin Sensitivity in Overweight Humans," *Diabetologia* 58, no. 10 (October 2015): 2324–35. https://doi.org/10.1007/s00125-015-3705-6.

39. Tyagi, V., et al., "Revisiting the Role of Testosterone: Are We Missing Something?: Semantic Scholar," January 1, 1970. https://www.semanticscholar.org/paper/Revisiting-the-role-of-testosterone:-Are-we-missing-Tyagi-Scordo/fc3fcc2587271aa7a3c0b3775bda0134e1948221.

40. Neuman, H., et al., "Antibiotics in Early Life: Dysbiosis and the Damage Done," *FEMS Microbiology Reviews*, U.S. National Library of Medicine, July 2018. https://pubmed.ncbi.nlm.nih.gov/29945240/.

41. McLaren, Rodney A., Fouad Atallah, and Howard Minkoff, "Antibiotic Prophylaxis Trials in Obstetrics: A Call for Pediatric Collaboration," *AJP Reports*, U.S. National Library of Medicine, April 2020. https://pubmed.ncbi.nlm.nih.gov/32309017/.

42. Kalghatgi, Sameer, et al., "Bactericidal Antibiotics Induce Mitochondrial Dysfunction and Oxidative Damage in Mammalian Cells," *Science Translational Medicine*, U.S. National Library of Medicine, July 2013. https://pubmed.ncbi.nlm.nih.gov/23825301/.

43. "Ciprofloxacin Has Dramatic Effects on the Mitochondrial Genome," *ScienceDaily*, October 1, 2018. https://www.sciencedaily.com/releases/2018/10/181001101943.htm.

44. Stefano, George B., Joshua Samuel, and Richard M. Kream, "Antibiotics May Trigger Mitochondrial Dysfunction Inducing Psychiatric Disorders," *American Journal of Case Reports*, International Scientific Information, Inc., January 7, 2017. https://www.amjcaserep.com/abstract/index/idArt/899478/act/2.

45. Shan, Jiang, et al., "Antibiotic Drug Piperacillin Induces Neuron Cell Death through Mitochondrial Dysfunction and Oxidative Damage," *Canadian Journal of Physiology and Pharmacology*, U.S. National Library of Medicine, July 31, 2017. https://pubmed.ncbi.nlm.nih.gov/28759731/.

46. Liu, Zhigang, et al., "Gut Microbiota Mediates Intermittent-Fasting Alleviation of Diabetes-Induced Cognitive Impairment," *Nature News*, Nature Publishing Group, February 18, 2020. https://www.nature.com/articles/s41467-020-14676-4.

47. Manyi-Loh, Christy, et al., "Antibiotic Use in Agriculture and Its Consequential Resistance in Environmental Sources: Potential Public Health Implications," *Multidisciplinary Digital Publishing Institute*, March 30, 2018. https://www.mdpi.com/1420-3049/23/4/795.

48. Becattini, Simone, et al., "Antibiotic-Induced Changes in the Intestinal Microbiota and Disease," *Trends in Molecular Medicine* 22, no. 6 (2016): 458–78. doi:10.1016/j.molmed.2016.04.003.

49. Samsel, Anthony, and Stephanie Seneff, "Glyphosate, Pathways to Modern Diseases III: Manganese, Neurological Diseases, and Associated Pathologies," *Surgical Neurology International*, Medknow Publications & Media Pvt Ltd, March 24, 2015. https://www.ncbi.nlm.nih.gov/pmc/articles/PMC4392553/.

50. Mesnage, Robin, et al., "Shotgun Metagenomics and Metabolomics Reveal Glyphosate Alters the Gut Microbiome of Sprague-Dawley Rats by Inhibiting the Shikimate Pathway," *bioRxiv*, Cold Spring Harbor Laboratory, January 1, 2019. https://www.biorxiv.org/content/10.1101/870105v1.

51. "Global Glyphosate Study by The Ramazzini Institute." Accessed September 13, 2020. https://glyphosatestudy.org/.

52. Martinez, Adriana, and Abraham Jacob Al-Ahmad, "Effects of Glyphosate and Aminomethylphosphonic Acid on an Isogeneic Model of the Human Blood-Brain Barrier," *Toxicology Letters*, U.S. National Library of Medicine. Accessed September 13, 2020. https://pubmed.ncbi.nlm.nih.gov/30605748/.

53. Peixoto, Francisco, "Comparative Effects of the Roundup and Glyphosate on Mitochondrial Oxidative Phosphorylation," *Chemosphere*, January 2006. Accessed September 13, 2020. https://www.researchgate.net/publication/7504567_Comparative_effects_of_the_Roundup_and_glyphosate_on_mitochondrial_oxidative_phosphorylation.

54. Juo, Chang-Hung, et al., "Immunomodulatory Effects of Environmental Endocrine Disrupting Chemicals," *Kaohsiung Journal of Medical Sciences*, U.S. National Library of Medicine. Accessed September 13, 2020. https://pubmed.ncbi.nlm.nih.gov/2287 1600/.

55. Petersen, Kate S., "Microplastics in Farm Soils: a Growing Concern," *EHN*, August 31, 2020. https://www.ehn.org/plastic-in-farm-soil-and-food-2647384684.html.

56. Juo, Chang-Hung, et al., "Immunomodulatory Effects."

57. "EWG's 2020 Guide to Safer Sunscreens," EWG. Accessed September 13, 2020. https://www.ewg.org/sunscreen/report/the-trouble-with-sunscreen-chemicals/.

58. Bosman, Else S., et al., "Skin Exposure to Narrow Band Ultraviolet (UVB) Light Modulates the Human Intestinal Microbiome," *Frontiers*, October 7, 2019. https://www.frontiersin.org/articles/10.3389/fmicb.2019.02410/full.

59. Oliveira, Karen Jesus, et al., "Thyroid Function Disruptors: from Nature to Chemicals," *Journal of Molecular Endocrinology*, Bioscientifica Ltd, January 1, 2019. https://jme.bioscientifica.com/view/journals/jme/62/1/JME-18-0081.xml.

60. Mikulic, Matej, "OTC Drug U.S. Retail Revenue 1965[en dash]2019," *Statista*, July 22, 2020. https://www.statista.com/statistics/307237/otc-sales-in-theus/.

61. Welu, Jenna, et al., "Pump Inhibitor Use and Risk of Dementia in the Veteran Population," *Federal Practitioner*, June 2019. https://www.researchgate.net/publication/334446750_Proton_Pump_Inhibitor_Use_and_Risk_of_Dementia_in_the_Veteran_Population. https://www.ncbi.nlm.nih.gov/pmc/articles/PMC6604981/.

62. Stoker, Megan L., et al., "Impact of Pharmacological Agents on Mitochondrial Function: A Growing Opportunity?" *Biochemical Society Transactions* 47, no. 6 (2019): 1757–72. https://doi.org/10.1042/bst20190280.

63. Lukić, Iva, et al., "Antidepressants Affect Gut Microbiota and Ruminococcus Flavefaciens Is Able to Abolish Their Effects on Depressive-like Behavior," *Nature News*, Nature Publishing Group, April 9, 2019. https://www.nature.com/articles/s41398-019-0466-x.

64. "News from #AAIC19: Surprising Differences Found in How Sleep Medications

Increase Dementia Risk for Some, Protect Others," AAIC. https://www.alz.org/aaic/releases_2019/monSLEEP-jul15.asp.

65. Hochuli, Michel, et al., "Sugar-Sweetened Beverages with Moderate Amounts of Fructose, but Not Sucrose, Induce Fatty Acid Synthesis in Healthy Young Men: A Randomized Crossover Study," *OUP Academic*, Oxford University Press, June 1, 2014. https://academic.oup.com/jcem/article/99/6/2164/2537861.

66. Jaiswal, N., et al., "Fructose Induces Mitochondrial Dysfunction and Triggers Apoptosis in Skeletal Muscle Cells by Provoking Oxidative Stress," *Apoptosis* 20 (2015): 930–47. https://doi.org/10.1007/s10495-015-1128-y.

67. *The Lifestylist Podcast*, "The Deep Science of Blue Light Toxicity, and Why LED Trashes Your Health with Dr. Alexander Wunsch," Episode 278. https://www.lukestorey.com/lifestylistpodcast/the-deep-science-of-blue-light-toxicity-why-led-trashes-your-health-with-dr-alexander-wunsch-278.

68. Pannala, Venkat R., Amadou K. S. Camara, and Ranjan K. Dash. "Modeling the Detailed Kinetics of Mitochondrial Cytochrome c Oxidase: Catalytic Mechanism and Nitric Oxide Inhibition." *Journal of Applied Physiology* 121, no. 5 (2016): 1196–1207. https://doi.org/10.1152/japplphysiol.00524.2016.

69. Russell, Cindy L., "5 G Wireless Telecommunications Expansion: Public Health and Environmental Implications," Environmental Research. U.S. National Library of Medicine, April 11, 2018. https://pubmed.ncbi.nlm.nih.gov/29655646/.

70. Bandara, Priyanka, et al., "Planetary Electromagnetic Pollution: It Is Time to Assess Its Impact," *Lancet Planetary Health* 2, no. 12 (December 2018): e512–14. doi:10.1016/S2542-5196(18)30221-3.

Chapter 7: The Energy Paradox Eating Program

1. Rosenbaum, Michael, et al., "Glucose and Lipid Homeostasis and Inflammation in Humans Following an Isocaloric Ketogenic Diet," *Obesity* (Silver Springs, MD), U.S. National Library of Medicine, June 2019. https://www.ncbi.nlm.nih.gov/pmc/articles/PMC6922028/.

2. Walton, Chase M., et al., "Ketones Elicit Distinct Alterations in Adipose Mitochondrial Bioenergetics," *MDPI*, August 29, 2020. https://www.mdpi.com/1422-0067/21/17/6255/htm.

3. Zhang, C., "The Gut Flora-Centric Theory Based on the New Medical Hypothesis of 'Hunger Sensation Comes from Gut Flora': A New Model for Understanding the Etiology of Chronic Diseases in Human Beings," *Austin Internal Medicine* 3, no. 3 (2018). https://doi.org/10.26420/austin-intern-med.2018.1030.

4. Zhang, Chenggang, et al., "Research Progress of Gut Flora in Improving Human Wellness," *Food Science and Human Wellness*, Elsevier, March 21, 2019. https://www.sciencedirect.com/science/article/pii/S2213453019300278.

5. Ma, Linqiang, et al., "Indole Alleviates Diet-Induced Hepatic Steatosis and Inflammation in a Manner Involving Myeloid Cell 6-Phosphofructo-2-Kinase/Fructose-2,6-Biphosphatase 3," *AASLD*, John Wiley & Sons, Ltd, June 29, 2020. https://aasldpubs.onlinelibrary.wiley.com/doi/abs/10.1002/hep.31115.

6. Wang, Dong D., et al., "Plasma Ceramides, Mediterranean Diet, and Incident Cardiovascular Disease in the PREDIMED Trial (Prevención Con Dieta Mediterránea)," *Circulation*, March 9, 2017. https://www.ahajournals.org/doi/10.1161/CIRCULATIONAHA.116.024261.

7. Meng, Xiao, et al., "Dietary Sources and Bioactivities of Melatonin," *Nutrients*, MDPI, April 7, 2017. https://www.ncbi.nlm.nih.gov/pmc/articles/PMC5409706/.

8. Murray, Andrew J., et al., "Dietary Long-Chain, but Not Medium-Chain, Triglycerides Impair Exercise Performance and Uncouple Cardiac Mitochondria in Rats," *Nutri-

tion & Metabolism, BioMed Central, January 1, 1999. https://nutritionandmetabolism .biomedcentral.com/articles/10.1186/1743-7075-8-55.

9. Bian, Xiaoming, et al., "Gut Microbiome Response to Sucralose and Its Potential Role in Inducing Liver Inflammation in Mice," *Frontiers in Physiology*, Frontiers Media S.A., July 24, 2017. https://www.ncbi.nlm.nih.gov/pmc/articles/PMC5522834/.

10. Yao, C. K., J. G. Muir, and P. R. Gibson, "Review Article: Insights into Colonic Protein Fermentation, Its Modulation and Potential Health Implications," Wiley Online Library, John Wiley & Sons, Ltd, November 2, 2015. https://onlinelibrary.wiley.com/doi /pdf/10.1111/apt.13456.

11. David, Lawrence A., et al., "Diet Rapidly and Reproducibly Alters the Human Gut Microbiome," *Nature*, U.S. National Library of Medicine, January 2014. https://pubmed .ncbi.nlm.nih.gov/24336217/.

12. Yao, C. K., et al., "Insights into Colonic Protein Fermentation."

13. Teigen, Levi M., et al., "Dietary Factors in Sulfur Metabolism and Pathogenesis of Ulcerative Colitis," *Nutrients*, MDPI, April 25, 2019. https://www.ncbi.nlm.nih.gov/pmc /articles/PMC6521024/.

14. Murray, Andrew J., et al., "Dietary Long-Chain, but Not Medium-Chain, Triglycerides Impair Exercise Performance."

15. Pinget, Gabriela, et al., "Impact of the Food Additive Titanium Dioxide (E171) on Gut Microbiota-Host Interaction," *Frontiers in Nutrition* 6 (2019). doi:10.3389/fnut.2019 .00057.

16. Peh, Meng Teng, et al., "Effect of Feeding a High Fat Diet on Hydrogen Sulfide (H_2S) Metabolism in the Mouse," *Nitric Oxide* 41 (2014): 138–45. https://doi.org/10.1016/j .niox.2014.03.002.

17. Park, Seonhye, and Yongsoon Park, "Effects of Dietary Fish Oil and Trans Fat on Rat Aorta Histopathology and Cardiovascular Risk Markers," *Nutrition Research and Practice*, Korean Nutrition Society and Korean Society of Community Nutrition, 2009. https://www.ncbi.nlm.nih.gov/pmc/articles/PMC2788173/.

18. Farajbakhsh, Ali, et al., "Sesame Oil and Vitamin E Co-Administration May Improve Cardiometabolic Risk Factors in Patients with Metabolic Syndrome: A Randomized Clinical Trial," *Nature News*, Nature Publishing Group, May 14, 2019. https://www .nature.com/articles/s41430-019-0438-5.

19. Marzook, Ebtisam A., et al., "Protective Role of Sesame Oil against Mobile Base Station-Induced Oxidative Stress," *Journal of Radiation Research and Applied Sciences*, No longer published by Elsevier, October 29, 2013. https://www.sciencedirect.com /science/article/pii/S1687850713000125.

20. Cienfuegos, Sofia, et al., "Effects of 4- and 6-h Time-Restricted Feeding on Weight and Cardiometabolic Health: A Randomized Controlled Trial in Adults with Obesity," *Cell Metabolism*, Cell Press, July 15, 2020. https://www.sciencedirect.com/science/article /pii/S1550413120303193.

21. Hara, Fumihiko, et al., "Molecular Hydrogen Alleviates Cellular Senescence in Endothelial Cells," *Circulation Journal*, Japanese Circulation Society, August 25, 2016. https://www.jstage.jst.go.jp/article/circj/80/9/80_CJ-16-0227/_html.

22. Phinney, Stephen, and Jeff Volek, "Sodium, Nutritional Ketosis, and Adrenal Function," *Virta Health*, January 2, 2020. https://www.virtahealth.com/blog/sodium -nutritional-ketosis-keto-flu-adrenal-function.

23. Abdelmalek, Manal F., et al., "Higher Dietary Fructose Is Associated with Impaired Hepatic Adenosine Triphosphate Homeostasis in Obese Individuals with Type 2 Diabetes," *Hepatology* (Baltimore, MD), U.S. National Library of Medicine, September 2012. https://www.ncbi.nlm.nih.gov/pubmed/22467259/.

24. Dewdney, Brittany, et al., "A Sweet Connection? Fructose's Role in Hepatocellular

Carcinoma," *Biomolecules*, U.S. National Library of Medicine, March 25, 2020. https://pubmed.ncbi.nlm.nih.gov/32218179/.

25. Baumeier, Christian, et al., "Caloric Restriction and Intermittent Fasting Alter Hepatic Lipid Droplet Proteome and Diacylglycerol Species and Prevent Diabetes in NZO Mice," *Biochimica et Biophysica Acta (BBA)—Molecular and Cell Biology of Lipids*, Elsevier, January 31, 2015. https://www.sciencedirect.com/science/article/pii/S1388198115000293.

26. Greenhill, Claire, "Benefits of Time-Restricted Feeding," *Nature News*, Nature Publishing Group, September 14, 2018. https://www.nature.com/articles/s41574-018-0093-2.

27. Cienfuegos, Sofía, et al., "Effects of 4- and 6-h Time-Restricted Feeding."

Chapter 8: The Energy Paradox Lifestyle

1.   Levine, James A., "Energy Expenditure of Nonexercise Activity," *American Journal of Clinical Nutrition* 72, no. 6 (2000): 1451–54. https://doi.org/10.1093/ajcn/72.6.1451.

2.   Kline, Christopher E., "The Bidirectional Relationship between Exercise and Sleep: Implications for Exercise Adherence and Sleep Improvement," *American Journal of Lifestyle Medicine*, U.S. National Library of Medicine, 2014. https://www.ncbi.nlm.nih.gov/pmc/articles/PMC4341978/.

3.   Carter, Heather N., Chris C. W. Chen, and David A. Hood, "Mitochondria, Muscle Health, and Exercise with Advancing Age," *Physiology*, May 1, 2015. https://journals.physiology.org/doi/full/10.1152/physiol.00039.2014.

4.   Memme, Jonathan M., et al., "Leg Exercise Is Critical to Brain and Nervous System Health," *ScienceDaily*, May 23, 2018. https://www.sciencedaily.com/releases/2018/05/180523080214.htm.

5.   Memme, Jonathan M., et al., "Exercise and Mitochondrial Health," The Physiological Society, John Wiley & Sons, Ltd, December 9, 2019. https://physoc.onlinelibrary.wiley.com/doi/abs/10.1113/JP278853.

6.   Severinsen, Mai Charlotte Krogh, and Bente Klarlund Pedersen, "Muscle-Organ Crosstalk: The Emerging Roles of Myokines," *OUP Academic*, Oxford University Press, May 11, 2020. https://academic.oup.com/edrv/article/41/4/594/5835999.

7.   Schmidt, W. D., C. J. Biwer, and L. K. Kalscheuer, "Effects of Long versus Short Bout Exercise on Fitness and Weight Loss in Overweight Females," *Journal of the American College of Nutrition*, U.S. National Library of Medicine, October 2001. https://pubmed.ncbi.nlm.nih.gov/11601564/.

8.   Murphy, M. H., and A. E. Hardman, "Training Effects of Short and Long Bouts of Brisk Walking in Sedentary Women," *Medicine and Science in Sports and Exercise*, U.S. National Library of Medicine, January 1998. https://pubmed.ncbi.nlm.nih.gov/9475657/.

9.   Hu, F. B., et al., "Walking Compared with Vigorous Physical Activity and Risk of Type 2 Diabetes in Women: A Prospective Study," *JAMA* 282, no. 15 (October 20, 1999): 1433–39.

10. Reynolds, Andrew N., "Advice to Walk after Meals Is More Effective for Lowering Postprandial Glycaemia in Type 2 Diabetes Mellitus than Advice That Does Not Specify Timing: a Randomised Crossover Study," *Diabetologia*, Springer Berlin Heidelberg, January 1, 1970. https://link.springer.com/article/10.1007/s00125-016-4085-2.

11. Kramer, Caroline K., Sadia Mehmood, and Renée S. Suen, "Dog Ownership and Survival," *Circulation: Cardiovascular Quality and Outcomes*, October 8, 2019. https://www.ahajournals.org/doi/10.1161/CIRCOUTCOMES.119.005554.

12. Allison, Mary K., et al., "Brief Intense Stair Climbing Improves Cardiorespiratory Fitness," *Medicine & Science in Sports & Exercise* 49, no. 2 (February 2017). https://journals.lww.com/acsm-msse/fulltext/2017/02000/brief_intense_stair_climbing_improves.10.aspx.

13. Bartholomae, Eric, et al., "Reducing Glycemic Indicators with Moderate Intensity

Stepping of Varied, Short Durations in People with Pre-Diabetes," *Journal of Sports Science & Medicine*, Uludag University, November 20, 2018. https://www.ncbi.nlm.nih .gov/pmc/articles/PMC6243616/.

14. Van Proeyen, K., et al., "Training in the Fasted State Improves Glucose Tolerance during Fat-Rich Diet," *Journal of Physiology*, U.S. National Library of Medicine, November 2010. https://pubmed.ncbi.nlm.nih.gov/20837645/.

15. Jeong, Jae Hoon, et al., "Activation of Temperature-Sensitive TRPV1-like Receptors in ARC POMC Neurons Reduces Food Intake," *PLOS Biology*, Public Library of Science, April 24, 2018. https://journals.plos.org/plosbiology/article?id=10.1371%2Fjournal .pbio.2004399.

16. Jeong, Jae Hoon, et al., "Activation of Temperature-Sensitive TRPV1-like Receptors."

17. Karimi, Sara, et al., "The Effects of Two Vitamin D Regimens on Ulcerative Colitis Activity Index, Quality of Life and Oxidant/Anti-Oxidant Status," *Nutrition Journal*, BioMed Central, January 1, 1970. https://nutritionj.biomedcentral.com/articles /10.1186/s12937-019-0441-7.

18. Bosman, Else S., et al., "Skin Exposure to Narrow Band Ultraviolet (UVB) Light Modulates the Human Intestinal Microbiome," *Frontiers*, October 7, 2019. https://www .frontiersin.org/articles/10.3389/fmicb.2019.02410/full.

19. Maruca, Matt, "Matt Maruca on Using Light to Improve Health: Wellness Mama Podcast," *Wellness Mama*, February 11, 2020. https://wellnessmama.com/podcast/matt -maruca/.

20. Wunsch, Alexander, "Video: Why the Sun Is Necessary for Optimal Health," UCTV, University of California Television, University of California, March 2, 2015. https:// www.uctv.tv/shows/Why-the-Sun-is-Necessary-for-Optimal-Health-29076.

21. Talalay, Paul, et al., "Sulforaphane Mobilizes Cellular Defenses That Protect Skin against Damage by UV Radiation," *Proceedings of the National Academy of Sciences*, U.S. National Library of Medicine, October 30, 2007. https://pubmed.ncbi.nlm.nih .gov/17956979/.

22. Pullar, Juliet M., et al., "The Roles of Vitamin C in Skin Health," *Nutrients*, MDPI, August 12, 2017. www.ncbi.nlm.nih.gov/pmc/articles/PMC5579659/.

23. Society for the Study of Ingestive Behavior, "Blue Light at Night Increases the Consumption of Sweets in Rats," *ScienceDaily*. Accessed September 28, 2020. www.scienc edaily.com/releases/2019/07/190709091120.htm.

24. Hauglund, Natalie L., Chiara Pavan, and Maiken Nedergaard, "Cleaning the Sleeping Brain—the Potential Restorative Function of the Glymphatic System," *Current Opinion in Physiology*, Elsevier, November 6, 2019. https://www.sciencedirect.com/science /article/pii/S2468867319301609.

25. Allison, Kelly C., and Namni Goel, "Timing of Eating in Adults across the Weight Spectrum: Metabolic Factors and Potential Circadian Mechanisms," *Physiology & Behavior*, U.S. National Library of Medicine, August 1, 2018, www.ncbi.nlm.nih.gov/pmc /articles/PMC6019166/.

26. Martinez-Lopez, Nuria, et al., "Autophagy in the CNS and Periphery Coordinate Lipophagy and Lipolysis in the Brown Adipose Tissue and Liver," *Cell Metabolism* 23, no. 1 (2016). http://www.sciencedirect.com/science/article/pii/S1550413115005240.

27. Hussain, Joy, and Marc Cohen, "Clinical Effects of Regular Dry Sauna Bathing: A Systematic Review," *Evidence-Based Complementary and Alternative Medicine*, Hindawi, April 24, 2018. https://www.hindawi.com/journals/ecam/2018/1857413/.

28. Masuda, A. et al., "The Effects of Repeated Thermal Therapy for Two Patients with Chronic Fatigue Syndrome," *Journal of Psychosomatic Research* 58, no. 4 (April 2005): 383–87. doi:10.1016/j.jpsychores.2004.11.005, https://pubmed.ncbi.nlm.nih.gov/1599 2574/.

29. Naumann, Johannes, et al., "Effects of Hyperthermic Baths on Depression, Sleep and Heart Rate Variability in Patients with Depressive Disorder: A Randomized Clinical Pilot Trial," *BMC Complementary and Alternative Medicine*, 1027, 17(1), 172. https://doi .org/10.1186/s12906-017-1676-5.

30. Househam A. M., et al., "The Effects of Stress and Meditation on the Immune System, Human Microbiota, and Epigenetics," *Adv Mind Body Med*, Fall 2017. https://pubmed .ncbi.nlm.nih.gov/29306937/.

Chapter 10: The Energy Paradox Supplement List

1. Bannai, Makoto, and Nobuhiro Kawai, "New Therapeutic Strategy for Amino Acid Medicine: Glycine Improves the Quality of Sleep," *Journal of Pharmacological Sciences*, 2012. https://pubmed.ncbi.nlm.nih.gov/22293292/.

2. Nicolson, Garth L., et al., "Clinical Uses of Membrane Lipid Replacement Supplements in Restoring Membrane Function and Reducing Fatigue in Chronic Diseases and Cancer," *Discoveries (Craiova, Romania)*, Applied Systems Srl, February 18, 2016. www.ncbi.nlm.nih.gov/pmc/articles/PMC6941554/.

3. Park, Jung Eun, P. B. Tirupathi Pichiah, and Youn-Soo Cha, "Vitamin D and Metabolic Diseases: Growing Roles of Vitamin D," *Journal of Obesity & Metabolic Syndrome*, Korean Society for the Study of Obesity, December 2018. https://www.ncbi.nlm.nih.gov/pmc /articles/PMC6513299/.

4. Hathcock, John N., et al., "Risk Assessment for Vitamin D," *OUP Academic*, Oxford University Press, January 1, 2007. https://academic.oup.com/ajcn/article/85/1/6/4649294.

INDEX

ABOUT THE AUTHOR

STEVEN R. GUNDRY, MD, is the director of the International Heart and Lung Institute in Palm Springs, California, and the founder and director of the Center for Restorative Medicine in Palm Springs and Santa Barbara. After a distinguished surgical career as a professor and chairman of cardiothoracic surgery at Loma Linda University, Dr. Gundry changed his focus to curing modern diseases via dietary changes. He is the author of the *New York Times* bestsellers *The Plant Paradox, The Plant Paradox Cookbook, The Plant Paradox Quick and Easy, The Longevity Paradox, The Plant Paradox Family Cookbook,* and *Dr. Gundry's Diet Evolution*; and the is host of the *Dr. Gundry Podcast*. He has published more than three hundred articles in peer-reviewed journals on using diet and supplements to eliminate heart disease, diabetes, autoimmune disease, and multiple other diseases. Dr. Gundry lives with his wife, Penny, and their dogs in Palm Springs and Montecito, California.